The Science of Occupational Health

The Science of Occupational Health: Stress, Psychobiology and the New World of Work

Ulf Lundberg and Cary L. Cooper

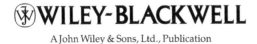

A John Wiley & Sons, Ltd., Publication

This edition first published 2011
© 2011 Ulf Lundberg and Cary L. Cooper

Blackwell Publishing was acquired by John Wiley & Sons in February 2007. Blackwell's publishing programme has been merged with Wiley's global Scientific, Technical, and Medical business to form Wiley-Blackwell.

Registered office
John Wiley & Sons Ltd, The Atrium, Southern Gate, Chichester, West Sussex, PO19 8SQ, United Kingdom

Editorial offices
9600 Garsington Road, Oxford, OX4 2DQ, United Kingdom
2121 State Avenue, Ames, Iowa 50014-8300, USA

For details of our global editorial offices, for customer services and for information about how to apply for permission to reuse the copyright material in this book please see our website at www.wiley.com/wiley-blackwell.

Wiley publishes its books in a variety of electronic formats: ePDF 9781444391107; oBook 9781444391121; ePub 9781444391114

Library of Congress Cataloging-in-Publication Data

Lundberg, Ulf.
   The science of occupational health : stress, psychobiology, and the new
world of work / Ulf Lundberg and Cary L. Cooper.
       p. ; cm.
   Includes bibliographical references and index.
   ISBN 978-1-4051-9914-8 (pbk. : alk. paper)   1. Job stress. 2.   Industrial
hygiene. I. Cooper, Cary L. II. Title.
   [DNLM: 1. Stress, Psychological–physiopathology. 2. Stress,
Psychological–prevention & control. 3. Occupational Health. 4. Socioeconomic Factors.
5. Workplace–psychology. WM 172 L962s 2011]
   RC963.48.L86 2011
   616.9'8–dc22

                                                                    2010022800
ISBN: 9781405199148

A catalogue record for this book is available from the British Library.

Set in 10/12pt Times by Thomson Digital, Noida, India.

1 2011

Contents

Foreword

Low-status people suffer from the ill-effects of work to a greater degree than do those of high status. Work is a contributor to social inequalities in health. That said, high-status people are not totally immune. The occupational hazard of being a king if Macbeth is one of your courtiers is abrupt shortening of life: death by dagger. Memorably, the drunken porter in Macbeth is the light relief between the murder of the King and the dire consequences of the tragedy that is Macbeth's, and Lady Macbeth's, malignant ambition. Light relief, perhaps, but wise words. The porter speaks of alcohol as an equivocator. I have adapted the porter's insight to describe alcohol as an equivocator with health – good and bad consequences. The same could be applied to work: an equivocator with health. Work can be life enhancing both as a positive force and as means to avoid the negative – the disastrous psychological and physical health consequences of unemployment. Yet bad work can be a potent cause of ill-health.

A recent WHO report estimated that 2 million people die each year as a result of work-related illnesses and injuries. Further, there are 268 million non-fatal work accidents annually. As a telling picture of the psychological toll of work, it has been estimated that 8% of the global burden of disease from depression is currently attributed to occupational risks.

The Commission on Social Determinants of Health (CSDH)[1], which I chaired, was informed by its knowledge network on employment and working conditions. Attention was drawn to the health effects of employment conditions and to the nature of the employment contract (if such exists), as well as to the nature of work itself. On a global scale, employment conditions are highly relevant. In developed economies, such as those within the European Union, about 85% of those in employment are wage and salary workers. About 10% are 'own account workers' or 'contributing family workers'. By contrast in South Asia and sub-Saharan Africa, fewer than 25% are wage and salary workers and about 75% are own account or contributing family workers. Such work, largely in the informal economy, is precarious, both in working conditions and in susceptibility to loss of employment.

The research on the health effects of work, admirably brought together in this book, has been gathered largely from high-income countries where, compared with what is happening elsewhere, we have had a high degree of attention to both employment conditions and the health effects of work, with regulation, health and safety legislation, occupational health services and much discussion on the nature of management for the well-being and productivity of workers. All of these findings are likely to apply, even more intensely, to the great swathes of the world's working population who are in the informal economy. The figures cited above for deaths and illness come only from formally registered workplaces. The true global figure will be very much higher. Work is an absolutely key health issue.

Another issue claims our attention. Both in CSDH, and in the Review of Health Inequalities in England (*Fair Society, Healthy Lives*)[2] for which I was responsible, we emphasised the simple issue of the need to organise our economic arrangements so that all in society have the minimum income necessary for a healthy life. Work, of course, is one route to achieving that minimum income level. Not outside the high income countries, however: in 2007, the CSDH reported, 1.3 billion workers did not earn above $2 a day.

Globally we have a kind of double burden in relation to work. The term 'double burden' has been applied to the fact that in low-income countries there is a heavy toll of both communicable and non-communicable diseases at the same time. Similarly, in low–middle income countries there is a double burden of under-nutrition and over-nutrition. Adapting this concept we could say that in high-income countries, as the physical conditions of work have improved, increasingly it is psychosocial hazards that account for illness related to work. Additionally, work is a route out of poverty and, at least in principle, a means of self-actualisation, of fulfilling one's goals and role in life. Indeed it is frustration of these wider purposes of work that are likely to be responsible for much physical and mental harm.

The double burden applied to work signifies that in low-income countries the issue of physical and biological hazards of work is far from solved. Nor is work necessarily a route out of poverty. Additionally all the adverse effects of psychosocial hazards apply as well.

Because the adverse effects of work and employment tend to be seen more frequently the lower people are in the social hierarchy, work is potentially a potent contributor to inequalities in health within and between countries. The CSDH called for the issue of health inequity to be part of the climate change/sustainability agenda. *Fair Society, Healthy Lives* echoed that call. As this book makes clear, a changing world has profound effects for the nature of work and its likely health effects. We need to be striving hard to make sure that the modern world of work, globally, is one that enhances human capabilities and is good for health. Similarly we must be striving to ensure that the nature of work and employment is good not just for us as individuals, but for society and for the planet. Surely, just as we must be thinking 'health and flourishing' when we think of work, so must we be thinking 'green'.

This book is a model example of how to bring to bear the best scientific evidence on a most important set of policy issues.

Professor Sir Michael Marmot
University College London
London

NOTES

1 CSDH (2008) Closing the gap in a generation: health equity through action on the social determinants of health. Final Report of the Commission on Social Determinants of Health. World Health Organization, Geneva.
2 Marmot Review (2010) *Fair Society, Healthy Lives: Strategic Review of Health Inequalities in England Post 2010*. Marmot Review, London.

Preface

In each new generation people have felt that they were born and live in a very special period in human history, and that conditions during their lives are changing more rapidly than ever before. Old products, techniques, ideas and values are replaced by new ones at an accelerating speed. If this is true, every new generation is indeed exposed to a faster pace of life than previous generations. Why, then, should we be concerned about the ongoing changes in working life today, and their future consequences? Is there something special going on today, compared with what earlier generations have experienced?

Yes, we think there is. Earlier major occupational changes, such as the Industrial Revolution and the introduction of assembly-line work, and the invention of new means of transport and communication such as railways, automobiles, telephones and aeroplanes, have had a great impact on people's lives, but this happened gradually. It took a rather long period of time until large groups of people were able to use and benefit from these facilities.

An important reason why we think that recent decades have been exceptional is the electronic revolution, which has changed people's lives dramatically in less than a generation. The first personal computers appeared only about 30 years ago. An ordinary PC today is much cheaper and at the same time more than 10 000 times as efficient in terms of speed and memory capacity compared with, for example, an IBM XT of the mid-1980s. This development made it possible for another even more dramatic electronic revolution, the introduction of the internet, which started only about 20 years ago and now influences people's lives in almost all countries all over the world. The internet provides access to immediate information on almost any subject, and has created opportunities for international direct communication between almost all the peoples in the world, unless restricted by political or economic means. Parallel to the increased use of the internet, mobile phones have developed rapidly into what today are small computers, TVs, cameras and online news agencies. These developments in electronics and the miniaturisation of the equipment have had a profound influence on our working conditions and other parts of our lives in the most developed countries. Examples are an intensification of work and diversification of products, the opportunity to stay in constant contact with work and colleagues and the possibility of working in almost any place and at any time of the day. Another consequence is that information is spreading immediately from one place to another all over the world, with extensive economic, occupational, political, technical and social consequences. Examples are the spread of economic crises from one country to another, frequent reorganisations and the introduction of new products and services, more global and liberalised economies, and more flexible forms of work and employment.

In a large part of the world, traditional physical risk factors still represent the dominating health problems, and efforts to reduce and eliminate exposure to such conditions are still a major priority. In the emerging economies today, notably China and India, representing about a third of the world's population, major changes in working life still consist of people moving from farming to industrial manufacturing. In countries that were industrialised earlier, such as North America, Europe and Japan, the ongoing changes consist mainly of workers moving from manufacturing to knowledge-intensive and service-based work.

Conditions in the more developed countries are complex, and involve interactions between individual, organisational, societal and international processes. Modern working life presents opportunities for the improvement of our economies and health, as well as new health risks. Physical occupational hazards have been reduced, but an increase in mental and musculoskeletal disorders is substantial, particularly in young women and in socially and economically disadvantaged groups of people. In this book we describe general trends in the modern workplace and how individuals, organisations and societies are affected, positively and negatively, and consider how changes in health and well-being can be understood from a psychobiological perspective. On the basis of this knowledge, we believe that more healthy work conditions can be created, with considerable economic and public health benefits.

Among future challenges and threats influencing working life, of particular importance are social inequity in health, women's work, stress and health, the ageing populations of the developed world, the growing world population and the greenhouse effect with global warming and rising sea levels. Given the times in which we are living, it is important to remember the words of President Franklin Delano Roosevelt, which were spoken during the Great Depression of the 1930s:

> True individual freedom cannot exist without economic security and independence. People who are hungry and out of a job are the stuff of which dictatorships are made. The hopes of the Republic cannot forever tolerate either undeserved poverty or self-serving wealth.

Ulf Lundberg and Cary L. Cooper
Stockholm and Lancaster

Acknowledgements

This book was prepared while Ulf Lundberg was on sabbatical, 2009–2010. He also wants to thank his wife, Agneta, for practical and emotional support.

Cary L. Cooper would like to thank all his doctoral students over the years for helping him to develop the field of occupational stress.

Original illustrations by Urban Skytt (urban.skytt@gmail.com), Stockholm, Sweden.

1 Introduction: History of Work and Health

GENERAL BACKGROUND AND AIM

Having a paid job is, for most people and in most cases, a source of economic security, status, well-being and health. It gives meaning to lives, but it can sometimes be a mental and physical burden and a source of frustration, conflict, disappointment, mental and physical illness and even death. This dualism has been caught elegantly in the title of an article by Lennart Levi (1990): 'Occupational stress. Spice of life or kiss of death?'. Dr Levi is a Swedish pioneer in occupational stress research, and presently, at the age of 80, an active Member of Parliament. His article describes how work-related psychosocial stressors affect human health through emotional, cognitive, behavioural and physiological processes, as modified by situational and individual factors. He presents evidence for a causal relationship between work-related psychosocial stressors and the incidence and prevalence of occupational morbidity and mortality, and emphasises the need for a better understanding of work environment–stress–health relationships. In this book we will follow up on his aspirations in order to learn more about stress and health in modern work life in a rapidly changing world.

We will identify and describe ongoing trends in the modern workforce from a stress–health perspective, and will also speculate on health consequences of future workforce developments. On the basis of recent scientific evidence, positive as well as negative aspects of modern workforce conditions will be outlined and will be related to health outcomes. We will also describe the psychobiological mechanisms linking stressful work conditions to morbidity and mortality. Work-related health problems comprise subjective health complaints as well as more serious disorders such as burnout syndromes, depression, musculoskeletal and cardiovascular disorders, diabetes, metabolic syndromes, cognitive impairment, susceptibility to infections and sudden death. The concept of 'stress' is used in a broad sense, similar to its popular usage. However, different forms and aspects of stress, and some influential models of occupational stress, will be described and applied to specific occupational conditions.

During the last couple of decades, the workplace in the USA, Europe and some highly developed Asian countries has undergone major changes involving introduction of 'downsizing and outsourcing', 'lean and just-in-time' production, longer working hours and temporary and part-time employment (NIOSH, 2002; Peña-Casas & Pochet, 2009). These changes started as a result of the recession in the early years of the 1990s and increased

The Science of Occupational Health: Stress, Psychobiology and the New World of Work, first edition
By Ulf Lundberg and Cary L. Cooper. Published 2011 by Blackwell Publishing Ltd
© 2011 Ulf Lundberg and Cary L. Cooper

business globalisation. The impact on the psychosocial work environment has been higher workloads and greater time pressures ('fewer people doing more'), increased speed of change, less predictability, decreased job security and job loss, but also, more positively, some control over work pace and work methods, increased flexibility and responsibility, and more learning opportunities. There has also been a continuous increase in the number of women in the workforce, and more and more dual-earner and single-parent families have emerged (Lewis & Cooper, 2005). In addition, changed family structures and increased care responsibilities for both children and older relatives have added to the pressures on large groups of workers in the industrialised and emerging world.

A consistent trend in a large part of the globe is that stress-related disorders are becoming more prevalent and severe (Cooper *et al.*, 2009). Stress may exert its health effects in different ways. It affects bodily functions and organs, such as the cardiovascular, metabolic and immune systems. Stress also influences people's lifestyles, for example their dietary habits, physical activity, and alcohol and tobacco consumption. In addition, stress can increase risk-taking behaviour, causing accidents at work and in people's private lives. Stress is also known to have negative effects on people's compliance with treatment regimens, such as taking prescribed medication to reduce high blood pressure or follow-up dietary recommendations for diabetics. Another indirect consequence is that stress can make workers less likely to use protective devices on the job, such as helmets, hearing protection and seat belts, or to follow instructions about how to use dangerous equipment in a safe way. The World Health Organization (2001) identified mental health problems and stress-related disorders as 'the biggest overall cause of early death in Europe'. According to the European Working Conditions Survey 2006 (Parent-Thirion *et al.*, 2007), 30–40% of workers reported such problems, with the highest figures in the new member states (Fig. 1.1). In the UK, stress has been estimated to cost the economy between 5 and 10% of GNP per annum (Fig. 1.2; Cooper, 2005). Mental illnesses (e.g. depression, chronic fatigue syndrome, anxiety, personality disorders, drug abuse problems, schizophrenia) and pain problems are the most common reasons for individuals describing their state of health as 'poor'. In Sweden these disorders are

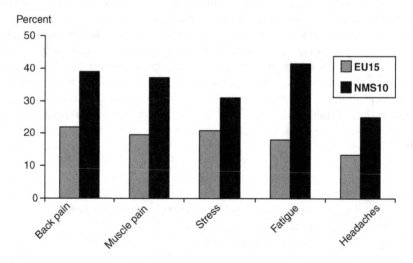

Fig. 1.1   Work-related health problems within the EU, 2006 (Parent-Thirion *et al.*, 2007). EU15 = Old 15 EU members. NMS10 = 10 new EU member states, 2006.

The costs of workplace stress and mental health problems

- Total cost to employers of mental ill health at work is ~ £29.5 billion per annum (1)
- Stress from work per annum costs employers ~ £3.7 billion (2)
- 13m working days are lost (3)
- Total cost of incapacity benefit per annum is £12 billion (4)
- Nearly 40% of people drawing IB have a mental health condition = £5 billion

  Cost of stress in the workplace results from wide range of sources such as:
  Sickness absence
  Labour turnover
  Premature retirement
  Health insurance
  Treatment of consequences of stress

  (1)   Sainsbury Centre for Mental Health (2008)
  (2)   CBI (2005)
  (3)   HSC (2004)
  (4)   DWP (2006)

  Government Office for Science, DIUS

Fig. 1.2   The costs of workplace stress and mental health problems in the UK.

responsible for 76% of sick-leave pay in women and 65% in men. In recent years it has been shown that psychosocial factors play an important role not only in mental, cardiovascular and metabolic disorders, but also in infectious diseases and in pain-related problems such as neck, shoulder and back pain, headache and stomach ache (as will be described in the following chapters). Recent research has revealed some of the psychobiological mechanisms involved in these relationships, although there is still a need for more research (Sapolsky, 1998; McEwen & Lasley, 2002).

Researchers from University College London have monitored workers' feelings about their job, recorded their heart rate and its variability, measured the stress hormone cortisol (see Chapter 5), and studied diet, exercise, smoking and drinking habits. They found that chronic work stress was associated with coronary heart disease, particularly in men and women under 50. This is consistent with results from the Inter-Heart Study (Yusuf *et al.*, 2004), a large investigation comprising 52 countries with about 15 000 cardiac patients and 14 000 controls in which the roles of different risk factors for chronic heart disease were evaluated. Next to cigarette smoking, psychosocial stress was found to be the most important risk factor for heart disease, increasing the risk almost three times (Fig. 1.3).

A deeper understanding of the processes involved in these trends and relationships is necessary in order to take measures to prevent work-related stress and ill health. The overarching goal of this book is therefore to present evidence on the ongoing trends and expected future developments in the workforce, and to describe the consequences for employees' mental and physical health. The aim is to highlight the new workplace in a modern and changing society, its various stress-related aspects and health consequences, future perspectives and possible preventive strategies. Empirical investigations, and theoretical and methodological developments in psychobiological stress research during the last decades, have provided new information on how mental processes affect various bodily functions such as the cardiovascular, immune and metabolic systems, the brain and the muscles (Sapolsky, 1998; McEwen & Lasley, 2002). However, it is important to keep in mind that physical occupational health risks are still a major health problem in a large part of the

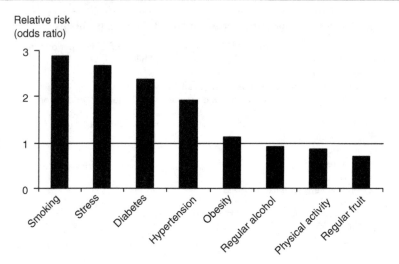

Relative risk
(odds ratio)

Fig. 1.3   Psychosocial stress (depression, locus of control, perceived stress, life events) and other risk (and protective) factors for myocardial infarction. INTERHEART case-control study (52 countries: 15 152 patients, 14 820 controls). Based on Yusuf *et al.* (2004) with permission.

world. According to the International Labour Organization (2005) about 2.3 million men and women, mostly in the developing world, die from work-related accidents and diseases each year, including an estimated 650 000 deaths caused by hazardous substances. These numbers are likely to be underestimated owing to the inadequate reporting and notification systems in many countries.

WORK AND HEALTH FROM AN EVOLUTIONARY PERSPECTIVE

It is now more than 200 years since the birth of Charles Darwin and over 150 years since the publication of his *On the Origin of Species*. It is therefore appropriate to look back on the role of 'work' in human history. The first modern human beings, *Homo sapiens*, appeared about 150 000–200 000 years ago. Their main 'job' was to gather edible plants, nuts, fruit and roots, and to hunt animals for food in order to survive and to be able to mate and multiply. It has been estimated that the first humans spent 2–3 days a week on finding food. This means an average daily 'workload' of 2 to 3 hours, which can be compared with about 8 hours or more of work as the norm today. As no artificial light was available, humans could not do anything else other than rest and sleep during the dark part of the day. Even after starting to use fire for heating and to create some light in the evening and during the night, a discovery that probably occurred about a million years ago in Africa among the ancestors of *Homo sapiens*, moving around in the darkness was difficult with a burning torch and, as a consequence, people tended not to move around much. As the only means of transportation was walking and running, the possibilities of moving longer distances were also limited by the nature of the landscape and because of threats from dangerous animals and hostile human beings. Today, however, humans can be more active, and move and travel around 24 hours a day thanks to electric lighting and more efficient means of transportation that can take travellers to almost any part of the world within a day or so.

Among animals the amount of time spent on their 'job' of finding food varies a great deal. Some birds spend almost all the time awake on finding food, whereas predators such as lions and tigers spend most of their time relaxing in the shade and only seek prey when they are hungry. Koalas are famous for spending most of the day asleep and only about 5 hours a day munching eucalyptus leaves. A large snake such as a boa constrictor can swallow a large animal and survive on this for months. Thus, from an evolutionary perspective, working 8 hours or more a day for survival is not genetically 'natural'.

Humans eventually found that farming and domestication of animals were more efficient means to guarantee a constant supply of food that made it possible for more people to live together and not have to move constantly to new places to find food. This meant that the workload increased considerably. Sowing seed, caring for crops and animals and harvesting made it necessary for people to work actively on a daily basis. Until the beginning of the 20th century and industrialisation, life as a farmer was the most typical job, and involved both women and men. Also children had to be mentally and physically active on a daily basis from an early age. Technological advances in the late 19th and early 20th centuries, such as the development of more productive seeds and of machinery for seeding and harvesting, combined with the introduction of more efficient methods including the use of fertilisers, reduced the need for manpower and decreased the physical demands to some extent. This did not, however, reduce the workload as more and more people moved into other jobs and activities, for example industrialised manufacturing.

Living close together with other people and with livestock increased the risk for transmitting infectious diseases such as upper respiratory infections, pneumonia and tuberculosis. The accumulation of waste in highly populated areas also contributed to health risks. As a consequence, health began to decline in humans in Europe about 3000 years ago. This was reflected in, for example, changing height in humans, which in men was reduced from about 173 cm around 400 BC to 166 cm in the 17th century. Not until the mid 19th century did health begin to improve. In recent decades lifestyle factors such as cigarette smoking, lack of physical activity and increasing overweight in affluent societies have caused worse health in large groups of people. Examples are lung cancer (due to cigarette smoking), which increased in men 20–30 years after starting to smoke and which is still increasing in women who started to smoke later, and Type 2 diabetes (due to overweight, stress, and lack of physical exercise), which is presently increasing in a large part of the developed and developing world. So far, however, life expectancy has continued to increase in most parts of the world thanks to better nutrition, sanitary improvements, better maternal and infant care, medical advances and improved treatments. For example, lowering blood pressure and blood lipids by medication combined with lifestyle changes have helped reduce the prevalence of cardiovascular disease (e.g. heart attacks, stroke) in the working population during recent decades. An exception to this trend of increasing life expectancy is Russia, where life expectancy decreased after the collapse of the Soviet Union.

For thousands of years, humans spread from Africa to other parts of the world. This process was very slow, and generation after generation lived under relatively similar and stable conditions. Around a thousand years ago, however, human cultures started to appear that were founded on more advanced methods and tools, specialisation in work techniques and the formation of larger and more organised societies. During the last two millennia, the speed of change has increased at an accelerating pace. For the last 100 years, societies and living conditions have changed dramatically and the speed of change appears to be continuing to accelerate, yet human beings as biological organisms have remained the same for a hundred millennia.

Humans are very flexible and are usually able to adjust to new demands and conditions with no, or only minor, short-term health problems. Within moderate limits, exposure to new conditions is likely to promote individual development, strength, health and well-being. However, there are limits to adaptation. In the late 1960s science journalist Alvin Toffler wrote *Future Shock* (Toffler, 1970) in which he described the accelerating speed of change and the pace of daily life in modern society. Toffler identified how changing lifestyles, and technological developments such as advances in transport and communication, were giving rise to new products, the rebuilding of city centres, the construction of shopping malls, and ever-larger streets and highways. Travelling within countries and abroad, moving home and changing jobs were all occurring more and more frequently. In addition, social relationships changed dramatically, with the extended family structure gradually disappearing. Toffler's aim was to analyse the personal and psychological, social and health consequences of accelerating change in society. He stressed that humans were about to reach a critical point at which they would be overwhelmed by change and would face a massive adaptational breakdown.

Toffler's fear of adaptational breakdown was based partly on research findings at that time by two psychiatrists, Thomas Holmes and Richard Rahe (1967). They constructed the Social Readjustment Rating Scale in order to measure the time and effort necessary to adjust to various life changes: 'the cost of adaptation'. Positive as well as negative events were included. This scale was based on normative ratings from a panel of individuals, giving weight to various possible events in an individual's life. Marriage was used as a standard and given a value of 50 (Fig. 1.4). Death of a spouse was rated as one of the most stressful events and given a value close to 100. By adding the weightings associated with each event during a specific period in life, a total life-change score could be calculated for single individuals. In several studies this score was related to cardiovascular events and it was found that an accumulation of life changes often preceded heart attacks and sudden deaths. The assumption behind this scale was that not only did negative events, such as death and sickness in the family, divorce and job loss, contribute to the 'cost of adaptation', but also positive events, such as marriage, having a new child, moving to a new home or starting a new job, would tax the individual's coping resources and take a toll that could be reflected in increased vulnerability and health problems. The new notion that positive changes can tax an individual's coping resources is supported by anecdotal evidence from individuals who suffered a heart attack just after they learned that they had won a fortune on the lottery or experienced some other kind of sudden dramatic positive event such as the unexpected survival of a loved one after a serious accident or a natural disaster. This suggests that sudden intensive positive emotions could trigger a heart attack in susceptible individuals, but strong scientific evidence for this phenomenon is difficult to find or obtain as controlled experiments are not possible for obvious practical or ethical reasons.

The Social Readjustment Rating Scale has since been modified, and the general assumption is that adjustment to new conditions as such is not a health problem provided that the individual also has sufficient time to prepare and to adjust to the new situation. Unexpected life events are more harmful for health than expected events, and negative events are more harmful than positive events. Events initiated by the individual him- or herself have also been found to be less harmful than events caused by external conditions or individuals.

In his book Toffler (1970) points out a number of future 'shocking' scenarios: babies born without pregnancy, cities under the sea, man–machine sexual relationships, sunshine at will, homosexual family units, antisocial leisure cults, accelerated education through drugs, animal servants and group marriages. As we can see today, 40 years later, some of these

Life event	Life change units
Death of a spouse	100
Divorce	73
Marital separation	65
Imprisonment	63
Death of a close family member	63
Personal injury or illness	53
Marriage	50
Dismissal from work	47
Marital reconciliation	45
Retirement	45
Change in health of family member	44
Pregnancy	40
Sexual difficulties	39
Gain a new family member	39
Business readjustment	39
Change in financial state	38
Change in frequency of arguments	35
Major mortgage	32
Foreclosure of mortgage or loan	30
Change in responsibilities at work	29
Child leaving home	29
Trouble with in-laws	29
Outstanding personal achievement	28
Spouse starts or stops work	26
Begin or end school	26
Change in living conditions	25

Fig. 1.4   Social readjustment rating scale (adults).

'shocking' predictions have come true but are not today considered very shocking. Indeed the speed of change in society has accelerated far beyond what Toffler had imagined. As an example of how family structures have changed, having children without being formally married (cohabitating) has become common in many countries. In countries such as Estonia and Sweden today, more than 50% of children are born outside formal marriage. In Nordic countries, about 50% of all couples separate at least once in life, and a 'modern' family today often consists of a couple with children from previous marriages and from their present relationship: 'my children, your children, our children'. Other examples of 'new families' today are single-sex families with and without children, which have become more frequent and accepted; children that are born after *in vitro* fertilisation; and single mothers with children born after insemination with sperm from an unknown father. The electronic revolution, with personal computers, the internet, email and mobile phones, could not be predicted in the 1960s.

In recent decades we have seen great changes in working conditions in industrialised countries, related to a more global economy and modern communication technologies that have given rise to more competition, increased demands for speed, efficiency and productivity, the faster pace of work and more deadlines (Fig. 1.5). In the more recently developed countries, such as China, South Korea and India, these changes have been even more rapid

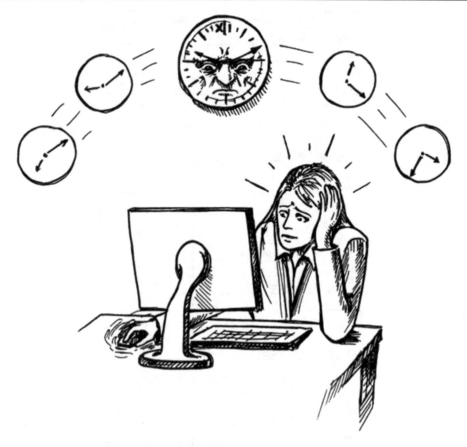

Fig. 1.5 Work pace is increasing. Drawing by Urban Skytt.

and dramatic, at least in the big cities. The development from life as a farmer to life in a computerised world took a hundred years for people in western countries but is now happening in a decade in China and India. This is likely to cause extra strain on people in these countries. In addition, repeated economic recessions, such as the most recent one that started in 2008, have contributed to additional turbulence and have intensified the restructuring of companies and manufacturing techniques, leading ultimately to reduction of personnel. Such changes will be followed by increased unemployment, and even higher demands on the remaining workers. Demands for more advanced training and education and a faster pace of work make it almost impossible for people without these qualifications to get a permanent job. There is a risk that many young people will fail to be part of the permanent workforce all their lives. In Sweden, for example, about 20% of the population in the 1950s had only primary education, and at that time about 20% of the jobs did not require additional training and education. Today, however, only about 5% of jobs can be performed by individuals without specific training and education, but more than 20% of each new generation lacks that kind of training or education. This means that about 15% of each new generation will not get a permanent job. An additional group of people who will face significant problems entering the workforce of the future will be people suffering from various health problems and handicaps. Immigrants without formal education, or with the 'wrong' sort of education from their homeland, also face significant difficulties finding a permanent job.

Millions of years of evolution created individuals who adjusted to conditions which differ dramatically from what humans are exposed to today. Evolution is a very slow process, and even minor biological changes via natural selection would take thousands of years. *Homo sapiens* has proved to be very flexible, and has been able to populate almost all parts of the world but has contributed to the extinction of other species. For more than a hundred thousand years, *Homo sapiens* and Neanderthals lived together on Earth but according to recent DNA research there was limited interracial mating. Around 30 000 years ago, Neanderthals disappeared and *Homo sapiens* remained as the only human species on Earth.

Despite the success of *Homo sapiens* on Earth, constant adjustment to rapidly changing and largely unpredictable conditions is likely to tax human resources. This may be one explanation for health problems reported today in industrialised countries. Although physical health has improved considerably in most parts of the world, as reflected in longer life expectancy and more children surviving their first year of life, mental health problems as reflected in stress and lifestyle-related disorders such as anxiety, depression, burnout syndromes, chronic fatigue, cognitive (memory) impairment, overweight, Type 2 diabetes, sleep problems and diffuse muscular pains have increased dramatically at the same time. Usually physical health problems lead to mental problems, and mental problems cause a deterioration in physical health. Therefore, better physical health reflected in increased life expectancy and poorer mental health seems to be a contradiction. This contradiction can be explained by the fact that improved physical health, often measured in terms of infant mortality and life expectancy, during the last few decades has resulted from medical improvements, regular medical check-ups, reduced cigarette smoking in Western societies, and better health information and nutrition. Poor mental health is a consequence mainly of psychosocial conditions but is usually not fatal. It is possible to live a long life and suffer from depressed mood and muscle pain. However, there are considerable health differences between countries. For example, a woman in Europe and Japan can expect to live until the age of 80 or more, whereas a woman in Africa has a mean life expectancy of less than 50 years.

Presently, the new forms of work are mainly represented in the most developed countries in Europe, North America, Australia and some Asian countries such as Japan and South Korea, but are found in many big cities all over the world. In large parts of the world, hazardous physical work conditions are still causing major health problems. Examples are coal mines in China and Russia; and exposure to poisonous chemicals in the manufacturing industry and to pesticides in farming in India, Africa and South America. However, as we have seen in other parts of the world, rapid development and a more global economy may also change conditions in these countries in the near future, and people may soon be exposed to the 'new forms of work' discussed in this book. In many industrialised countries that depend on automatised production and more people working in white collar jobs, it is likely that mental stress has become the most important health problem. This could partly be the result of a reduction in physical health risks, but also of increased psychosocial demands (Pejtersen & Kristensen, 2009).

The UK Government's Foresight Project on 'mental capital and wellbeing' (Cooper *et al.*, 2009) explored the challenges and opportunities facing the UK over the next 20 years and beyond in terms of its mental capital, defined as:

> the totality of an individual's cognitive and emotional resources, including their cognitive capability, flexibility and efficiency of learning, emotional intelligence and resilience in the face of stress. The extent of an individual's resources reflects his/her basic endowment

(genes and early biological programming), and their experiences and education, which take place throughout the lifecourse.

The project report identified the factors that impinge on the national mental wellbeing of the UK population. It focused on the challenges that lie ahead as a result of globalisation and associated increased demands for competitiveness, together with increased pressures on working lives and the disruption of work–life balance. Also identified were the challenges from changing family structures and care responsibilities, not only for children but also for older relatives. The increased life expectancy in most industrialised countries and an ageing population in Europe and Japan mean that larger numbers of people will be at risk of dementia and other neurodegenerative diseases. The pension crisis in many countries as a result of the recession and the collapse of the banking sector means that people will need to work longer with consequent implications in all societies.

ABOUT THIS BOOK

First we will describe the new workplace and its characteristics in a rapidly changing world, and its positive and negative effects (Chapters 2–4). Then we will present scientific evidence on the conditions at work that are 'health promoting' as opposed to 'health damaging'. We will summarise from a psychobiological perspective the bodily effects of stressful work conditions, and the mechanisms that link these effects to various disorders. Possible interventions to reduce stress and promote health and productivity will be described on an individual, organisational and societal level. Gender and socioeconomic differences in work-related stress and health will be of particular interest in view of the fact that women generally report more symptoms than men, and that in affluent societies low-status individuals have more health problems and a shorter lifespan than high-status individuals. Finally, we will summarise the main conclusions and speculate about future perspectives on work as it relates to health.

2 The New Workplace in a Rapidly Changing World

GLOBAL ECONOMY AND GLOBAL COMPETITION

During the last few decades, political and economic changes in a large part of the world, and in Europe and the European Union (EU) in particular, have created increased competition not only between companies within a country but also between countries. Capital and production have become more mobile, and companies move their plants to countries and areas where the production costs are lowest. Workers also move between countries, but so far, only 4% of EU citizens have ever moved to another country in the EU and less than 3% to another country outside the EU (European Commission, 2007). Movement of capital and workers between countries is desirable from many points of view, and has been stimulated by the European Monetary Union (EMU) and a common currency, the euro. Also EU countries not part of the EMU are strongly influenced by the value of the euro. A free movement of workers, capital and companies within the EU has contributed to more competition and has made it possible for less developed countries with lower personnel costs to compete with more advanced countries in terms of services and goods. Private companies have always been exposed to competition, but with a more global economy and more liberal economic policies the competition has been intensified and has also involved competition from companies in other countries. Furthermore, what used to be the public service sector, run by local authorities or governments and financed via taxation, has also been exposed to competition from private enterprises. This may explain why the increase in stress-related disorders that occurred during the 1990s was particularly dramatic among people working in schools, hospitals and nursing homes, who were used to being protected from competition and from the risk of becoming redundant and of losing their jobs.

At the same time there has been a shift from industrial and manufacturing work towards more people being involved in 'knowledge-intensive' work with information and communications technology (Castells, 1996–2000; Cortada, 1998; Burton-Jones, 1999; Paganetto, 2004) and in the service sector. The shift away from manufacturing to work in the service sector has reduced exposure to many health hazards (Peña-Casas & Pochet, 2009). According to the European Foundation for the Improvement of Living and Working Conditions (2005; Parent-Thirion et al., 2007), 66% of workers in the 25 EU states were employed in the service sector, and the proportion of workers who use computers at least a quarter of the time has increased, from 31% in 1991 to 47% in 2005. There has also been a shift away from more simple to more 'qualified' work demands, and a reduction in personnel without formal education and training. To some extent employees with more 'qualified' educational backgrounds have had to take over the work tasks from those who have had to leave. One example is in hospitals, where licensed nurses and medical doctors have a much greater administrative burden compared with 15 years ago and, as a consequence, have less time for the patients and more conflicting demands at work. In most countries, the demands for more 'qualified' tasks and intensified work demands have not been compensated by giving workers more opportunities for learning and training at work, particularly among older people. In addition, more work is carried out in shifts and without fixed schedules, and health-related absenteeism has increased. In the 12 new member states of the EU, older women (age 55 +) are most subject to chronic illness as a result of these changes.

In several European countries, a new development during the 1990s was that the public service sector became more liberalised and exposed to competition from private companies. Examples are education, caring work (hospitals, dentistry, care of children and the elderly), the supply of electricity and water, transportation (buses, railways) and telecommunications (telephone, television, radio). Many of these companies are now privatised and compete with each other and with organisations that are still part of the public service sector. For individuals who have been employed by the government or local government without competition from other actors, the present situation is often perceived as more demanding and insecure. In Sweden, for example, schools, medical and elderly care, electricity and telephone companies, railways, radio and television were mainly run by the government or local government on a non-profit basis until the beginning of the 1990s. After a serious economic crisis in Sweden in the early 1990s, and after becoming a member of the EU, considerable restructuring and reorganisation of private and public companies, and a free movement of capital between countries, were introduced in order to increase competition, efficiency and productivity. In addition, technical and medical advances reduced the number of beds in hospitals, and length of treatment diminished. For example, in the 1970s, mothers used to stay in the maternity ward for up to a week after childbirth. Today, most mothers return home on the same day or the day after their child is born. Better medication, less invasive surgery ('keyhole' surgery) and computerisation have helped reduce the time spent at hospital. This has also meant that care-givers have a shorter time with each patient, and 'patient turnover' has increased. The number of less qualified care-givers has been reduced in favour of trained nurses and medical doctors, which has reduced the time for personal contact between patients and care-givers. Treatment has also become more 'medicalised' and technical as a result of new drugs and electronic developments.

A similar but less rapid and dramatic development occurred in many other countries. With the increase in international communication via electronic means such as email and the internet, changes and new developments in one part of the world rapidly spread to other parts including big cities in the generally less developed countries in the world. The reduction in personnel and increased demands for education and special competencies made large groups of workers redundant, and unemployment increased. A knowledge of foreign languages and of how to handle computers and advanced technological and electronic equipment, an understanding of written instructions, and mathematical and statistical skills became necessary in most jobs. Being a slow worker, lacking experience and education or having health problems increased the risk of losing one's job, or of not being able to enter the workforce at all. Workers were laid off and young people had difficulties getting into the

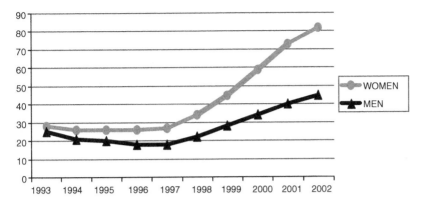

Fig. 2.1   Number of people on long-term (more than one year) sick leave in Sweden 1993–2002 (thousands).

labour market. In summary, this created polarisation, with increased work demands and overstimulation for some groups of workers, and lack of work and understimulation for other groups. This also increased socioeconomic differences between groups. Although the mean standard level of living increased, rich people became richer (and healthier), whereas the economic standard of the poor and their health increased very little. In countries such as Sweden, Norway and The Netherlands, these changes in the labour market at the beginning of the 1990s were followed by a dramatic increase in sickness absence and long-term absenteeism in particular. For example, in Sweden one-year absenteeism or more increased 200% for men and 300% for women from 1997 to 2002 (Fig. 2.1). The most common diagnoses were musculoskeletal disorders (MSD) such as neck, shoulder and back pain, and psychological problems, such as chronic fatigue, burnout syndromes, sleep problems and stress.

Changes in sick leave in the 1990s differed considerably between European countries. There are several reasons for this. Generally, sick leave is not a good measure of health in different countries. It depends on the proportion of different types of workers (for example, manual workers versus white collar workers), on the proportion of female workers, and the type of work. Some jobs can be performed even when the worker has health problems. The rules and regulations for economic compensation, and the right to keep the job during sick leave, also differ between countries. In countries such as Sweden it has until recently been possible to be on sick leave for several years and, at least formally, to have a job to return to. In other countries, Denmark, for instance, people who are ill for a longer period of time lose their job and are registered as 'unemployed' rather than on 'sick leave'. This makes comparison of trends in sick leave between countries a very crude and unreliable measure of health.

FLEXIBLE ORGANISATIONS – FLEXIBLE WORKERS

In order to meet the demands of the global economy and of an increasingly diverse market, companies and organisations have to become more flexible. One way to do this is to create more flexible forms of employment, such as temporary and part-time employment and the use of support from the employment services industry. For example, within the EU, temporary employment increased from 10% in 1991 to 14% in 2005 and part-time employment from 13% to 19% (Parent-Thirion *et al.*, 2007). A more adaptable workforce is required to help companies to survive.

New recruitment or interim management companies have been created in order to offer trained personnel, for example medical doctors, nurses, teachers and skilled manual workers, to other companies and organisations and to hospitals and schools on a short-term basis. This has made it possible to adjust the number of workers to current needs and to production demands, and to maintain only a small part of the workforce in permanent employment. This means more flexibility for the organisation, but creates more uncertainty and insecurity among the workers. Sora *et al.* (2009) examined the influence of an 'insecurity climate' on about 1000 employees' job attitudes in Spain and Belgium. The results showed that job insecurity decreased employees' job satisfaction and organisational commitment above and beyond individual perceptions of job insecurity. Artazcoz *et al.* (2005) reported that poor mental health among manual workers in Spain increased from about 5–10% among workers with a permanent job to 25–30% in workers with no job security. Kivimäki, Vahtera *et al.* (2003) presented evidence indicating that mortality is significantly higher among temporary workers compared with permanent workers.

A larger proportion of temporary jobs also increases the demands on permanently employed workers. Hired temporary workers can focus on their main task, for example, doctors and nurses can take care of and treat patients whereas their colleagues in permanent employment also have to take care of administrative work and make strategic and economic decisions, for example deciding when it is necessary and economically justified to engage extra personnel. In addition, workers from employment services companies are usually better paid than their permanently employed colleagues but sometimes have less education and experience, which can contribute to conflicts in the workplace. In some cases workers who have left their employment return or continue to work at their previous workplace but with another employer and a higher salary. The permanently employed workers also have to prove themselves within the company in order to stay employed, which could make them less willing to complain about bad working conditions and unfair treatment. Thus, external manpower support can also, to some extent, increase the burden on permanent staff.

According to a recent national study of the development of the psychosocial work environment in Denmark from 1997 to 2005 (Pejtersen & Kristensen, 2009), deterioration is seen in all subgroups of employees. In their study not only did work pace increase but it was also found that conflicts at work, slander and gossip increased, and negative relationships were found in respect of role conflicts, role clarity and lack of social support. According to the authors 'the observed negative trends should be interpreted in light of the development of the globalised economy and the new trends in the public sector such as new public management' (p. 291). In addition they conclude that 'increased competition and rate of changes together with the rapid introduction of new management technologies may well lead not only to higher quantitative demands but also lack of predictability, lower meaning of work, loosening of social networks, more job insecurity, and decreased role clarity' (p. 291). However, some positive trends were also seen such as increased quality of leadership and support from supervisors. Denmark is probably an example of a country with a rather good psychosocial work environment, characterised by the so-called 'flexicurity' model which means that high flexibility of the workforce is combined with high levels of security for the employees in terms of economic compensation during unemployment and sick leave. Pejterson and Kristensen (2009) point out that 'in spite of the political effort to improve the work environment, the overall tendency has been in the opposite direction' (p. 291). According to the National Institute of Occupational Safety and Health in the USA and European

Working Conditions Survey 2005, similar trends have also been seen in many other countries. The secondary analysis of the Fourth European Foundation for the Improvement of Living and Working Conditions (Parent-Thirion *et al.*, 2007) shows that the most unfavourable working conditions are seen in sectors such as agriculture, transport and construction and in hotels and restaurants, whereas people working in education, insurance and the financial sector enjoy a more favourable situation. A possible explanation for this trend is a shift away from manufacturing work to work in the service sector. This has reduced exposure to physical health hazards, but has increased work intensity.

HEALTH CONSEQUENCES OF 'SICKNESS PRESENTEEISM'

When permanently employed workers are reduced and have to take greater responsibility for daily business while feeling job-insecure, 'sickness presenteeism' may arise. Even when they feel ill, workers go to their job in order to show their employer that they are healthy, motivated and committed employees who show up every day. In job-insecure times, being 'present' is perceived to be a way of inoculating yourself against the next tranche of redundancies. Other reasons for going to work when feeling ill are that no one else can or will do the work that needs to be done, and/or that work tasks accumulate while the employee is absent from work, leading to extra stress and a heavier workload when he or she returns. Biron *et al.* (2006) investigated 9000 employees of a Canadian governmental organisation (response rate 51%), and found that a high workload increased presenteeism for employees. Another important reason for sickness presenteeism is of course the economic costs of being absent from work. In several countries, Sweden for example, no economic compensation is given for the first day off from work. The aim of this rule is to reduce short-term sickness absenteeism, assumed to be caused by minor health problems that are not necessarily a hindrance to work. Being able to take a day off from work when not feeling well, however, could contribute to a faster recovery and reduce the risk of long-term absenteeism (Kristensen, 1991). Furthermore, what may be considered a minor health problem in one group of employees may be a serious health problem in another and vice versa, depending on type of job and work tasks. For example, for an airplane pilot, a lorry or taxi driver, or a surgeon, feeling tired and having difficulties concentrating may cause a fatal accident whereas the same mental conditions are far less potentially harmful if you are a shop assistant or work in a supermarket. A scientist or an author might be able to work normally even with a broken leg, which would of course be impossible for a construction worker or a nurse.

From a short-term perspective, going to work when feeling unwell may be beneficial both for the company and for the employee. However, in the longer term, not responding to bodily signals means that minor health problems may develop into more serious health conditions. In a paper from the Whitehall study, Kivimäki, Head *et al.* (2005) assumed that male workers with no recorded days of absenteeism often tended to work when they were ill. These workers' risk of serious coronary disease was found to be twice as high as it was for those men who had a moderate amount of sick leave (1–14 days). This was considered to be evidence of a detrimental effect of 'sickness presence' as a result of the lack of recuperation in the group with no absences compared with those who had one or several days of absence. Hansen and Andersen (2009) collected information from a random sample of 11 838 members of the Danish workforce and found that sickness presence was associated with increased long-term sickness at a later date, even after controlling for a wide range of potential confounders as well as baseline health status and previous long-term sickness absence. In addition, going to

Table 2.1 Estimated annual costs to UK employers of mental ill health (Sainsbury Centre for Mental Health, 2007).

	Cost per average employee (£)	Total cost to UK employers (£ billion)	Per cent of total
Absenteeism	335	8.4	32.4
Presenteeism	605	15.1	58.4
Turnover	95	2.4	9.2
Total	**1035**	**25.9**	**100**

work with, for example, a common cold or influenza increases the risk that other people will be infected too and thus causes problems for them and, ultimately, bottom-line costs for the company. Biron *et al.* (2006) found that, on average, workers came to work 51.5% of the time they were ill. They also reported that workers with high levels of distress, and part-time and contractual workers, were more likely to work when ill than those with lower levels of distress and with permanent job status, respectively.

In the Sainsbury Centre for Mental Health (2007) report on the costs of stress and mental ill health sickness absence to the UK economy, you can see that (as shown in Table 2.1), the cost of presenteeism is nearly double the cost of absenteeism. This reflects the recession and increasing concerns about job security, forcing people to come to work even if they are ill and showing more 'face time' in the workplace, leading to a long-hours culture.

The effects of economic and occupational conditions on absenteeism can be illustrated by what happened in Sweden and some other countries in western Europe during the early 1990s. After the economic crisis at the beginning of the 1990s, which was followed by major reorganisations and reduction of personnel, absenteeism in Sweden decreased for some years despite consistent reports of increased stress and workload. Later during the 1990s, however, this trend was reversed and absenteeism from work increased drastically (Fig. 2.1). A likely explanation, supported by studies (e.g. Cooper & Dewe, 2008), is that after the economic crisis and the dramatic increase in unemployment, workers strained themselves to the limit of their capability in order to be as productive and competitive as possible and to be loyal to their organisation and to their colleagues, and appeared at work even when they felt unwell. Sickness presenteeism kept sickness absenteeism low for some years, but the combination of intensified workload and going to work when ill was followed by a dramatic increase in long-term absenteeism. A similar development can be expected as a result of the economic crisis that started in 2008. In summary, when fewer people have to do more and even go to work when they feel ill, this taxes their resources and will sooner or later cause longer term health problems. Uncertainty about having a job in the future, or about what future work tasks will look like, combined with economic strain, will increase experiences of stress both on and off the job and thus will lead to reduced opportunities for rest and recovery which are essential for long-term health.

RATIONALISATION

In continuous process manufacturing, the increased demands for efficiency and competition and the need to reduce costs are being met by rationalisation, automation and mechanisation. One example is that manual welding in the automobile industry has to a large extent been replaced by robots, which are faster and more precise and cost less than human welders. In addition, robotisation has reduced many health problems associated with welding, such as pain problems in arms and shoulders and exposure to smoke and heat. In this sector, production has been increased even without increasing demands on the remaining workers, and is associated with beneficial health consequences. However, this development has also meant that many qualified workers, such as welders and other skilled employees, lost their jobs and their status, leading to economic problems, distress, sleep difficulties and other health problems in these groups.

In the public service sector, such as teaching in schools, medical care in hospitals, care of children and the elderly and in many other service jobs, possibilities for rationalising work are much more limited. In these jobs increased competition and demands usually mean that people have to work faster, which in many cases influences not only their own situation but also the quality of their work, for example in providing less time to care for children and the elderly and for patients. This may explain why stress-related disorders and sickness absence in Sweden during the late 1990s increased most among people working in all of these caring professions.

In manual jobs that are difficult to automate, and where people cannot be replaced by robots, higher demands for productivity could increase the risk of accidents. Increasing work pace beyond an optimal level may not only increase the risk of health problems but may also be counterproductive from an economic perspective. Requests for additional increases in the pace of work may lead to a reduction in the quality of the product and in its value for the company. There are examples (J. Eklund, personal communication) that show that reduced work pace among cutters in the meat industry can save money for the company as more meat can be used from the animal and its quality is higher (there are fewer damaged pieces of meat).

The process of commercialisation of education, health care, water supply, electric power supply, public transport and other social arenas in recent decades has been combined with increased access to health-damaging commodities, such as fast high-fat foods, sugar and salty products, tobacco and alcohol, as the public service sector's possibilities for regulating the market have diminished. This contributes to increased health differentials between groups of individuals and countries. Those that have greater resources and power are more likely to be able to withstand this trend. The global and unregulated economy contributed to the banking crisis that started in 2008, which mainly affected groups with low socioeconomic status (for example in terms of lay-offs and increased income inequalities within and between countries).

SOURCES OF STRESS AT WORK

Cooper and Dewe (2008, p. 225) explained the background of how stress in the workplace has developed over the last 20–30 years.

> In the 1980s in the developed world we had the 'enterprise culture' (i.e. globalisation, greater competition, lean production), and in the 1990s and the early part of the first decade of the 2000s, we had the 'flexible workforce' (i.e. outsourcing, short term contracts). But, as we were to discover by the end of the 20th century, there were substantial personal costs for many individuals, as employees had to cope with constant change, job insecurity, heavier workloads and longer working hours. This 'cost' was

captured by a single word, 'stress'. Indeed, workplace stress has found as firm a place in our modern lexicon as 'texting', 'blackberrys' and 'junk bonds'!

These excessive pressures in many workplaces have been very costly not only to the individuals who suffered from stress but also to the bottom line of the businesses involved. The collective costs in the USA of organisational stress in all its manifestations (i.e. sickness absence, premature retirement due to ill health, etc.) have been estimated at $150 billion a year. In the UK, mental ill health and stress represent 40% of all incapacity benefit paid by the state, which is nearly £5 billion out of a total of £12 billion per annum. In addition, the employers' organisation and the professional body of personnel managers in the UK calculate the sickness absence costs per annum at £3.7 billion (Cooper & Dewe, 2008). None of this, however, takes into account the costs of presenteeism (where people turn up to work stressed and deliver little if any added value to their product or service), premature retirement due to mental ill health, and the costs to the health service of repairing the damage created by work (the last of which are likely to be enormous) (Dewe *et al.*, 2010).

The global world we live in has been strongly influenced by the US economy in the past 20 years, but the Far East (i.e. China and India) is likely to have more of an impact in the next two decades. The Americanisation of the workplace in Europe and elsewhere has meant leaner organisations in terms of employment, intrinsic job insecurity, a culture of long working hours, and a much more bottom-line management style focused on short-term results. This has meant that the 'psychological contract' between the employee and employer has truly been broken, with organisations demanding greater commitment, more flexibility from their point of view and longer working hours but not underwriting job security or demands for greater work–life balance by more truly flexible working arrangements. This trend in working life was reflected by the recent Quality of Working Life Survey carried out among a cohort of 10 000 managers (from shop floor to board level) by the UK's Chartered Management Institute. This found that nearly two-thirds of all organisations had introduced a 'cost reduction programme', 57% introduced the use of short-term contract staff and 25% had used outsourcing of various functions. These changes were perceived by managers at all levels as decreasing motivation (57%), and as leading to a reduced sense of job security (66%), poorer well-being (48%) and poorer morale (61%). It was also found that one in two managers did not feel positively motivated at work. Of those who felt motivated and had positive well-being, two out of three had higher productivity levels. In addition, 67% of managers who had suffered ill health and lack of mental well-being at work reported that it had reduced their individual productivity. When it came to management style, it was found that 40% of their senior managers were perceived as 'bureaucratic' and 30% as 'authoritarian', with only a few in the 'accessible and empowering' category. And finally, 89% of employees in this survey reported that they worked beyond their contracted hours every week, nearly two out of three saying these hours were damaging their relationship with their children, 59% their relationship with their spouse/partner, and 54% their health and productivity.

Change has been the byword of the first part of this millennium, with its job insecurities, major restructurings, overload and a significantly different and bottom-line management style. In other words, there has been massive organisational change and inevitable stress. The challenge for public and occupational health professionals in the future is to understand a basic truth of human behaviour: that developing and maintaining well-being at work is not just about higher salaries or increased productivity. It is, or should be in a civilised society, about quality-of-life issues as well, such as reasonable hours of work, manageable work-loads, control over one's job and career and some sense of job security.

Changes in the labour market have resulted in increased stress among large groups of the population. People in gainful employment have in general better health than whose who are not employed, but since the unemployed are a smaller group their influence on health in the population as a whole is of minor significance. In Sweden (Statistics Sweden, 2008), the proportion of women and men experiencing their work as both hectic and mentally taxing has increased since the 1980s, and has roughly followed the same trend as the incidence of stress symptoms. This trend was followed by an increase in sickness absence 1–3 years later. Workers in the public sector report that hectic and mentally taxing work increases during periods of recession, particularly among people who work in the health and educational sectors. In addition, teachers, and health and medical care staff, who often are women, are involved in work with other people. Such jobs are known to be 'emotionally demanding', and require people with good mental health.

Cooper and Marshall (1976) have described five major sources of stress at work:

1. Intrinsic factors, such as poor physical working conditions, work overload or time pressure.
2. Organisational role such as role ambiguity and role conflict.
3. Career opportunities, including job insecurity and under/overpromotion.
4. Poor relationships with boss and colleagues and/or bullying in the workplace.
5. Organisational structure and climate, including little involvement in decision-making and office policy.

These factors are part of the ASSET model (Faragher *et al.*, 2004), which also includes work–life balance, satisfaction from work, control and autonomy and levels of commitment to and from the organisation. On the basis of the ASSET stress questionnaire, 26 occupations were investigated with regard to work-related stressors and stress outcomes (Johnson, 2009). The six occupations that were found to be worse than average in terms of physical and psychological well-being and job satisfaction were ambulance workers, teachers, social services, customer services call centres, and prison and police officers. Johnson *et al.* (2005) have suggested (p. 184) that:

Each of the above occupations involve emotional labour, an element of work which has been described as relevant to the experience of work related stress in that all these job roles require either face to face or voice to voice interaction with clients, and in each of these occupations the emotions that the employees are required to display as part of their job have to follow strict rules. Think of, for example, the emotional labour that teachers have when working with unruly or unwilling to learn children without letting a child see their frustration, or the demands on police officers when facing potentially dangerous and volatile situations, whilst through necessity having to be outwardly calm and appear to be fully in control of a situation.

The least stressed and most satisfied occupations are analysts, school lunchtime supervisors and Directors/MDs within the private sector. Interestingly Directors in the public sector score higher on all three factors than Directors/MDs in the private sector although this finding is reversed when looking at management rather than Director level. Here, management in the private sector, score higher than management in the public sector on all three factors.

As part of the Quality of Working Life Project (Worrall & Cooper, 2007), large-scale research has been carried out on UK managers' work–life balance and psychological and physical health. It was found that from 2001 to 2006 an increasing number of managers had experienced more forms of change simultaneously, and that cost reduction was the prime driver of change. These changes increased the pressure on managers to work harder and longer. In 2007, 92% of managers in the UK regularly worked over their contract hours; the average amount of extra work was 1.47 hours per day. Working long hours had negative effects on their social life and reduced their opportunities for rest and recuperation, which is a key factor for health (see Chapter 9). In keeping with this, the majority of managers reported that the hours they worked over their contract hours had affected their health and well-being and had a negative impact on their relationships with their spouse/partner and children. Of 22 different stress factors in organisations, the following received the highest scores by the managers (Worrall & Cooper, 2007, pp. 138–139):

1. I have to deal with difficult customers/clients.
2. My work interferes with my home and personal life.
3. My pay and benefits are not as good as those of other people doing work similar to mine.
4. I do not have enough time to do my job as well as I would like.
5. I work longer hours than I choose or want to.
6. My performance at work is closely monitored.
7. I have little control over many aspects of my job.
8. My organisation is constantly changing for change's sake.
9. I may be doing the same job for the next 5–10 years.
10. I am given unmanageable workloads.
11. I am not involved in decisions affecting my job.
12. My job is adversely affecting my health.
13. I am set unrealistic objectives.
14. I spend too much time travelling in my job.
15. I have little or no influence over my performance targets.

It was concluded that (p. 144) 'despite all these actions to improve productivity and the large number of hours that managers gave free in the form of working over their contract hours, productivity in the UK remains below that of other main European competitors.'

A comparison between perceptions of managers in the UK ($n = 2451$) and in Victoria, Australia ($n = 1283$) (Worrall *et al.*, 2008) shows that there is great concern about the health risks associated with long working hours. The most frequently reported health problems in both countries were constant tiredness, muscular tension and insomnia, reported by about 60% of the respondents. Forty-five per cent of the respondents reported that their productivity at work was compromised as a result of the long hours spent on the job. Managers also felt that their social lives and personal relationships were negatively influenced by their long working week. In summary, it was found that Australian managers had a more positive view of their organisation, productivity and senior management compared with their UK colleagues. Possible explanations were that Australian managers, compared with UK managers, had a higher job satisfaction and had more trust in their management and felt more fairly treated and that targets and objectives were more realistic, and believed that they had better resources and that their organisation was more transparent and promoted well-being. The percentage of managers affected by organisational changes was higher in the UK, and changes in the UK were more often driven by cost reduction (59.5% in UK, 19.5% in Australia).

In terms of the impact of long working hours on health, as part of the prospective Whitehall II study of British civil servants, Virtanen *et al.* (2009) examined whether exposure to long working hours (more than 55 hours a week, compared with working 35–40 hours a week) predicts sleep disturbance. It was found that repeat exposure to long working hours was associated with a more than threefold increase in risk for shortened sleep, and an almost sevenfold increase in risk for difficulty in falling asleep. It was concluded that working long hours appears to be a significant risk factor for sleep disturbance.

3 The New World of Work

LEAN MANUFACTURING AND JUST-IN-TIME PRODUCTION

Until the beginning of the 1980s it was common in the manufacturing industry, for example in assembly work, to use 'buffer systems'. Different components of a product were produced independently of each other, and stored until needed. In a second step, the separate components were combined into a full product, for example a car engine, body parts, wheels, etc. and eventually a complete car. Under these circumstances a technical problem in the production line or a temporary lack of personnel was not a great problem, as a number of components were always available in stock. In addition, if the workers had already produced enough components, they could take a break. Even though the actual work tasks were specified and performed repeatedly, employees had some influence over their work flow and time pressure was reduced. It was quite common among assembly workers to work intensively for a certain period of time in order to be able to take a break and relax at other times.

In Sweden unscheduled 'coffee breaks' have, for a long period of time, been an accepted form of rest and an important social event in most workplaces, although the time is taken from paid work. A coffee break in the morning and at about 3 pm has been considered of great importance for job satisfaction, social cohesion and well-being among the employees, and probably also for productivity. In recent years, increased demands for efficiency, increased work flow and global competition, combined with reduced number of personnel, have made employers less supportive of this kind of paid rest.

Lean manufacturing and 'just-in-time production' aim at increasing efficiency and decreasing waste by optimising flow in order to increase competitiveness in the marketplace and ultimately the profits of the organisation. Anything that does not add value to the final product gets eliminated. In addition, the aim is to empower workers and enable production decisions to be made at the lowest level possible. Advantages include lower lead times, reduced set-up times, and lower equipment expenditure.

Just-in-time production strives to improve a business's return on investment by reducing inventory and associated costs. The process is a system of production that provides a signal for when a product should be manufactured, to produce only what is required in terms of quantity and at the right time. This means that stock levels of raw materials, components,

The Science of Occupational Health: Stress, Psychobiology and the New World of Work, first edition
By Ulf Lundberg and Cary L. Cooper. Published 2011 by Blackwell Publishing Ltd
© 2011 Ulf Lundberg and Cary L. Cooper

work in progress and finished goods can be kept to a minimum. Supplies are delivered right to the production line only when they are needed.

Advantages of just-in-time production are a reduction in storage space, which saves rent, insurance and personnel costs; there is less working capital tied up in stock; and there is less likelihood of stock perishing, becoming obsolete or out of date. Disadvantages are that there is little room for mistakes, and production is very reliant on suppliers. If stock is not delivered on time, the whole production schedule can be delayed and there are no spare products available to meet unexpected orders.

There are many similarities between just-in-time and lean production. Anything considered as 'wasteful' should be eliminated. This includes personnel, time and material not directly necessary for the goal of production. Inventory should be kept a minimum, only what is required being produced at the right moment.

A typical example of just-in-time and lean production is the assembly line in the automobile industry, where engines, wheels, seats and all parts to be combined with the body of the car are produced in parallel to be fitted to the rest of the car on the assembly line at the right time. A technical problem along the line or lack of personnel or supply would, in such cases, cause a complete stop in the production process, and a delay, which would be associated with enormous costs. Thus, this is not allowed to happen, and therefore workers have to compensate for such events by working more intensively or working extra hours to eliminate the delay and produce the necessary number of components planned for the day. Just-in-time production was also necessary to fulfil the requirements from customers to produce more personal products on demand. For example, automobiles today are often produced after an order from a customer, with personal specification of colour, model, type of engine, and other equipment in the car. This creates more variability for the assembly workers along the line, but also puts more pressure to fulfil the contract with the customer and meet the deadline of delivery compared with manufacturing products for stock.

Another example of this type of work is the checkout counter in a supermarket. Before competition increased in the early 1990s, cashiers working at the checkout counter who did not have any customers at a particular time could take a short break and chat with their co-workers. This opportunity is likely to increase social support and job satisfaction and contribute to rest and recovery from work. However, when competition increased, the companies decided to eliminate all 'natural breaks' and the checkout staff were requested to be constantly active. Personnel were therefore reduced to a minimum, and the number of open checkout counters was adjusted to fit the number of customers in the store. Companies required that there should always be a number of customers waiting in line to be served at the checkout counter. Expectations from the customers with regard to rapid service increased the stress of the work situation for cashiers. In order to keep staff busy, even when there were few customers in the store, more flexible work conditions were introduced by job rotation (Rissén *et al.*, 2002). Workers moved between different tasks depending on customer demands. For example, if there was a need for more cashiers at the checkout counters, workers had to be taken from other less urgent tasks at short notice to serve waiting customers. When there were few customers in the store, staff were requested to perform other tasks, such as filling the shelves, sorting out-of-date products, putting on price labels, and handling goods delivered to the store. This had some positive effects by creating more variability and responsibility in terms of work tasks, and a higher status among some of the workers (serving at the checkout counter is usually a low-status job in the supermarket), but at the same time increased uncertainty, time pressure and stress as workers had to move from one work task to another depending on where the demands at that moment were highest. The possibilities for social interaction with co-workers became limited, which is likely to have reduced job satisfaction. In addition, the introduction of job rotation was aimed at increasing productivity and was often combined with a reduction in the total number of employees (Rissén, 2006).

Although lean and just-in-time production has increased productivity and efficiency in many cases, there are certain risks associated with a very slimmed-down organisation, especially from a longer perspective. When employees are kept constantly active, there is very little time for reflection, problem solving or innovation, for future planning or for new ideas to emerge. In the longer term, this may cause a lack of renewal of products, services and methods, which could reduce the company's possibilities for competing and staying on top of the market in the future. All time, energy and concentration are focused on keeping the immediate production goals. Insufficient planning and renewal could make the company production obsolete and inefficient in the longer term. A very slimmed-down organisation also means that time for maintenance and repair of equipment is reduced, which could cause stoppages in the production, unnecessary delays and considerable costs for the organisation in terms of health, good will and economy. In addition, as described above, speeding up work pace is not always associated with increased productivity and economic benefits as the quality of the products may decline.

However, according to a study on 1391 workers at 21 sites in four UK industry sectors, lean production as such is not necessarily stressful (Conti *et al.*, 2006). Stress levels were found to depend very much on management policies and practices. Lean production may eliminate wasteful time and improve performance and quality of work, and thus generate pride and a sense of job security. The relation between lean implementation and job stress was found to be described by an inverted U-function. Initially, implementation is associated with increasing stress, then stress levels off. In the advanced stages of lean production implementation, stress decreases as a result of improved project efficiency, improved quality, more orderly workplaces and more predicable flow. However, lack of time for rest and recovery could still be a problem for long-term health. On the basis of the Karasek Work–Demand–Support Model (see Chapter 4), Conti *et al.* (2006) concluded that high work load and low social support were more strongly related to stress than control in lean production.

FREQUENT RESTRUCTURING

In order to adjust to new and more rapidly changing technical, political, social and economic conditions and to respond to requests for new products and services with an ever shorter lifespan, companies and organisations have to reorganise more often than before. Reorganisations and restructuring are also often performed in order to improve work conditions, productivity and health, but still require workers to adjust repeatedly to new demands and new conditions. Reduced exposure to pollution, noise and bad ergonomic conditions is of course positive from a health perspective. However, such changes, if initiated by the company without the informed participation of the employees, may also create feelings of uncertainty about what will happen next, what the employees are expected to do, who will be their boss and their co-workers in the future, etc. Also, the adjustment to positive changes requires time and energy and therefore taxes the individual's coping and adjustment resources. As demonstrated in the 1970s by Holmes, Rahe and others (e.g. Holmes & Rahe, 1967), and as mentioned in Chapter 1, individuals with a high 'life-change score' according to the Social Readjustment Rating Scale are at increased risk of coronary heart disease and potential sudden death. Frequent reorganisations without employee engagement and participation also contribute to reduced well-being, more distress and impoverished relations between employees and employers (Bowles & Cooper, 2009). The first or even the second reorganisation may be perceived as positive by employees in improving working conditions, but when reorganisations become more and more frequent, negative reactions tend to dominate. Employees in organisations undergoing frequent change often suggest that they would prefer to stay in a less optimal organisation rather than to have to adjust repeatedly to new organisational cultures.

Organisational changes such as mergers and acquisitions (Cooper & Finkelstein, 2009) and outsourcings have been found to increase the risk of depression (Niedhammer *et al.*, 1998), and repeated downsizing or rapid expansion have been found to increase hospitalisation and long-term sickness absence (Westerlund *et al.*, 2004). Kivimäki, Vahtera *et al.* (2001) investigated musculoskeletal problems in 764 municipal employees working in Finland before and after an organisational downsizing. After adjustment for age, sex and income, major downsizing was associated with a significant threefold increased risk of severe musculoskeletal pain among those who remained in employment. The largest contribution came from increases in physical demands, particularly in women and low-income employees, but reduction of skill discretion and increased job insecurity also contributed to the association. Restructuring that occurs repeatedly within a short period of time seems to be particularly harmful. A deterioration of social relationships and engagement in a work environment, associated with restructuring, may be more important for people's health than the restructuring *per se* (Kivimäki *et al.*, 2000). An increasing number of employees feel that they are not being heard, and believe that repeated downsizing and restructuring adversely affect their opportunities to do good work, resulting in increasing frustration and ultimately ill-health.

Reorganisations usually also involve replacement of senior management in order to bring new competence, ideas and methods into the organisation. This also means that managers and staff do not have time to learn about each other and how to collaborate. Frequent reorganisations often reduce opportunities for social relations, which are important for work satisfaction, productivity and health. Clear and efficient leadership is very important for good performance, social relations and well-being, whereas conflicts, negative mood and insufficient social support owing to lack of knowledge about the organisation and weak emotional relationships between workers and management have a negative impact on productivity and health. Middle management has been abandoned in many companies in order to create a more 'flat' organisation, under the assumption that this will make communication more efficient. A negative consequence of this is that workers do not know whom to talk to when they need help, and the emotional distance between workers and management becomes too great. Communication between workers and management therefore becomes limited, and significant problems in production and in relationships on the shop floor may exist without being noticed by management. In organisations in which workers feel insecure, they are also less likely to complain about bad working conditions.

LIFELONG LEARNING, WORK AND FAMILY-LIFE BALANCE

From a life-course perspective, the effects of changing work conditions may interact with changes in other parts of life. Childcare responsibilities and care for the elderly or sick relatives are demands that may reduce opportunities for people to find a new job, to engage more in paid work and lifelong learning and to take managerial responsibilities. Today, people in the western industrialised countries wait longer before having their first child. In Sweden, for instance, parents are around the age of 30 when they have their first child. One reason for this is that people have longer education years and cannot afford or have not enough time to take family responsibilities as long as they are studying. This also means that each new generation will have older parents, who may have their own health problems and be in need of care and attention rather than being a resource for their children and grandchildren.

Hence, many parents have just got or are looking for their first job when their first child is born. Demands from a recently started occupational career have to be combined with the demands of finding and creating a home for the family and taking care of small children. The costs of buying and furnishing a new home, financing the purchase of a car and its maintenance and paying off loans may cause economic strain. Individuals' opportunities to handle this situation depend very much on their social situation and political policies regarding family support, taxation and access to and costs of child day care. Parents often have to make a choice regarding how to balance their finances, family time and occupational career. The number of children with only one parent (usually the mother) at home has also increased in western countries. Single parents' resources to balance work and family life are of course particularly limited, and may explain their more frequent health problems and higher absenteeism from work.

Opportunities for maternal and paternal leave differ between countries. In Sweden, for instance, parents are allowed one year's paid maternal or paternal leave when a child is born, and a guaranteed return to their former job as long as the company or organisation is in business. In the United States, conditions are quite different and a quick return to work is usually necessary not only for economic reasons but also in order not to lose one's job. Among American first-time mothers employed during pregnancy and giving birth between 1996 and 2000, 60% had returned to work within 3 months after delivery. This means that paying attention to personal and work factors that promote women's health and successful return to work is of particular importance.

Full-time employment is usually necessary for parents to secure a reasonable economic living, especially when they have entered the labour market late in life and have student loans to pay off. Full-time employment is usually also necessary for future career opportunities, more skilled jobs and a higher income in the future. As pension at retirement is often based on income during active working life, full-time employment is also important for economic resources after leaving the paid workforce.

Working part-time will give more time for family matters, but will negatively affect the family's finances and future career opportunities. Many women but very few men choose to reduce their paid work hours or stop working when they have small children in order to decrease conflicts between paid and unpaid work demands, giving priority to childcare and housework. One reason for this gender difference is, of course, traditional gender roles, according to which the man is the breadwinner and the woman is responsible for childcare and household duties. According to the European Foundation for the Improvement of Living and Working Conditions (2005), women in the EU countries spend almost twice the amount of time as men on caring for children, the elderly and people with dependent needs. However, among dual-career full-time-employed parents, women also take a much greater share of childcare and domestic work and responsibility compared with men (Lundberg & Frankenhaeuser, 1999). In all countries within the EU except Austria and Germany a higher proportion of women than men feel that they do more than a fair share of housework (European Quality of Life Survey, 2003). In Sweden, women's average work hours in gainful employment have increased every year since the 1980s. Between 1979 and 2005, mothers with small children (up to the age of six) increased their work hours from an average of 27 to 34 hours a week, whereas fathers decreased theirs from 41 to 39 hours. In contrast to northern Europe, where women's part of the labour force is similar to that of men, less than 50% of women in southern Europe have a paid job. However, women's participation in the labour market is increasing in all countries. For example, in the US labour force, participation rates have changed from 31% in 1976 to 55% in 2004 for mothers of infants (child under one year of age). This means that gainful employment is taking up more and more of parents' time in families with small children, and that women's increasing engagement in paid work is not balanced by a corresponding increase in men's responsibility for childcare and unpaid work at home.

Lifelong learning with re-education, various flexible working options and different forms of employment contracts create more possibilities for learning and flexibility but also mean greater insecurity. In order to identify variables mediating the effects of role stressors on job performance, Fried *et al.* (2008) performed a meta-analysis of studies conducted over a period of 25 years. Data from 113 independent samples with more than 22 000 individuals were analysed. It was found that psychological and attitudinal variables were of importance for the relationship between role stress and job performance. More specifically, it was found that role stress was both directly and indirectly related to job performance through job satisfaction and propensity to leave. The mediating role of job satisfaction for job performance and propensity to leave was emphasised, and it was concluded that increasing job satisfaction is useful in order to reduce stress.

LONG WORKING HOURS AND OVERTIME

Generally, long working hours and overtime work are associated with health problems (Van der Hulst, 2003; Caruso *et al.*, 2004; Burke & Cooper, 2007). Two possible mechanisms for this relationship have been suggested: effects of high workload on psychophysiological functions and on health-related behaviours. Long working hours activate bodily functions such as blood pressure, heart rate and secretion of stress hormones over long periods of time and allow little time for rest and recovery. For example, Park, Kim, Chung *et al.* (2001) investigated subjective fatigue in South Korean men working less than 60 hours per week, between 60 and 70 hours, and more than 70 hours, and found a significant relationship between complaints of subjective fatigue and long working hours. As described in Chapter 5, long-term imbalance between activation and rest/recovery will exhaust bodily systems and cause dysregulation of important functions, as reflected in mental and physical symptoms and illness such as depression, chronic fatigue, burnout, sleep problems, pain syndromes, infections, and gastrointestinal disorders (ulcers, irritable bowel syndrome). Furthermore, lack of time for recuperation and sleep may induce compensatory effort of bodily stress systems to avoid deteriorating performance and thus cause additional load on these functions.

During periods of long working hours and excessive overtime, health-related behavioural changes may take place. There is less time for regular physical activity, and one may choose an unhealthy diet of fast food based on too much fat and sugar. Cigarette smokers under work-related stress are likely to smoke more. The need to smoke is one of the few more accepted reasons for taking a break, and hence smokers tend to smoke more in order to get a chance to take a break. Just taking a break because you feel the need to relax from the pressure of work is generally not considered appropriate. Alcohol consumption may increase during work overload since taking a drink after work makes it easier to relax mentally but not necessarily physiologically because of the effects that alcohol has on blood pressure and heart rate. Alcohol may also be used to reduce depressive feelings, at least in men. Men's greater consumption of alcohol may partly explain the gender difference in antidepressant medication. Women more often use antidepressant medication than do men, whereas men tend to use alcohol as the 'medicine of choice' against depressive symptoms.

These two mechanisms, changes in physiological arousal and behavioural changes towards a more unhealthy lifestyle, separately and in combination are two possible ways in which long working hours may cause health problems. In addition, tiredness/fatigue associated with long working hours could also cause an increased risk of accidents. A review of overtime work in 22 countries (Stier & Lewin-Epstein, 2003) suggests that preferences for work were affected by both individual and country-level factors, and that there was an overall preference to reduce overtime work.

Excessive overtime is usually associated with ill health (Beckers, 2008), but there is no linear or simple relation between workload and health problems. Even employees with a very high workload can be healthy (Krantz et al., 2005), but health status in these groups tends to differ between men and women and according to the type of job. For example, it has been shown that women regularly working more than 10 hours extra each week have a significantly increased risk of dying from heart attack compared with women's normal risk (Alfredsson et al., 1985). Men in the same situation have a reduced risk of heart attacks compared with men's normal risk. One likely explanation for these contrasting findings is that women working overtime usually have a larger responsibility for childcare and unpaid work tasks at home compared with men and therefore have less time for rest, recovery and recuperation. Men with small children and full-time employment, particularly in high status jobs, often have a part-time working partner taking care of unpaid work at home. This is seldom the case for women in the same position. Another possible explanation is that men and women have different positions in working life, and that men have a greater influence over whether and when they work extra hours whereas women more often are ordered to work overtime and have no choice. This difference in influence or control over the work situation between women and men also has consequences for circumstances outside work. A woman will have to manage others in the family to handle the domestic arrangements when she is not there as a result of staying late or working extra hours. For men, especially when they can choose themselves, working extra hours in the evening may be more relaxing as they can finish their work tasks without time pressure, and when they come home they can relax because dinner is ready and the children are in bed – all done by the woman!

One possible explanation for the fact that even a rather high workload is not necessarily associated with health problems could be that one has to be very healthy in order to regularly work 50 hours or more per week: 'reversed causation'. However, when the combination of paid and unpaid work becomes extremely high, influence and control decrease and health problems become more common for both women and men. Children contribute to increased total workload for both parents (Lundberg et al., 1994), but more so for women than for men. Children also have different effects on men's and women's paid workload. For women, there is a negative relation between number of children and hours in paid work. For men, there is a positive relation between number of children and paid work hours up to three children, then men start to reduce their workload slightly. For men, more flexible arrangements do not necessarily mean that they take a greater responsibility for household activities and childcare.

Virtanen et al. (2009) examined the association between long working hours and cognitive function in middle age in a prospective study of 2214 British civil servants (Whitehall II), who were in full-time employment at baseline. A battery of cognitive tests were performed at baseline and at follow-up five years later. Working more than 55 hours per week, compared with 40 hours or less, was associated with lower scores in the vocabulary test at both baseline and follow-up. Long working hours also predicted decline in performance on a reasoning test. The results remained after adjustments for age, sex, marital status, education, occupation, income, physical diseases, psychosocial factors, sleep disturbances, and health risk behaviours, and show that long working hours may have a negative effect on cognitive performance in middle age.

In a field survey of 238 male engineers in three electronics manufacturing companies in South Korea (Park, Kim, Cho *et al.*, 2001), measures of cardiovascular functions (blood pressure, heart rate variability) and self-reports of working hours, health conditions and fatigue were obtained. Overtime work was found to be related to cardiovascular functions. Low frequency component of the heart rate variability during work was considered as an early objective indicator for chronic effects of regular overtime work on cardiovascular functions.

THE ROLE OF MODERN COMMUNICATION TECHNOLOGY AND TELECOMMUTING: WORK WITHOUT BOUNDARIES, OR ENDLESS WORK

Mobile phones, emails, laptops and the internet have made it possible for many employees to keep in constant contact with their work. It is possible to work from home, and while travelling, staying in hotels and eating in restaurants and so on. As this opportunity exists, it is often expected from employers, managers and colleagues that the employee will be available by phone almost 24 hours a day and will respond promptly to emails and SMS even when off work, such as in the evening and during weekends and holidays. This gives employers more control over their employees and their work activities. Such expectations are likely to interfere with other parts of life of the employee, such as family life, leisure activities and rest. At the same time, this form of flexibility gives the worker more freedom to work when it is suitable without having to be present at the workplace.

With modern communication technology it is possible to work almost 'without boundaries' in time and space (Allvin *et al.*, 2011). As work tasks in many jobs today are unspecified and goal oriented, it is up to the employee to decide how much time and effort to devote to work, and even how work should be defined. Without a specific work environment, physical and organisational improvements in the workplace are not always relevant for the employee's work situation. Such jobs, where the employee has great responsibilities, unclear work tasks and significant mental demands, are mostly found among upper-level public employees (Kristensen *et al.*, 2002). These groups of employees experience increased stress symptoms. This may be due to increased work requirements in recent years, which have not been compensated for by more influence over the work situation. Greater responsibility for defining their work assignments and for setting limits for the scope of their work and the overlap between work and other parts of life is likely to have contributed to higher mental demands. Individuals high in work commitment and with performance-based self-esteem are likely to be particularly vulnerable to such work outcomes.

Although most workers are still performing their job in a specific work environment with specific work conditions and colleagues and are starting and ending their work at specified hours, an increasing number of people, particularly within the 'knowledge intensive' sector, have few specified work tasks, workplaces or working hours. This trend is a consequence of increasing demands on companies to reach important short-term goals. Examples are a more rapid turnover and a greater customisation of products and services in the market. In addition, there is increased global competition, and the capital markets expect rapid pay-off (yield) of investments. This means that economic short-term output is prioritised compared with long-term financial goals.

Certain goals are to be reached and certain products are to be delivered to a customer, but it is up to the worker to decide how to reach these goals and how much time and effort should be put into this achievement. People working as consultants, journalists and other freelancers may also have to define their own goals and work tasks, and find out where to seek information, whom to collaborate with and when to finish the task. This means that the individual has to take on all responsibilities, and set the limits. In the service sector, and when working with other individuals, it may be difficult to set limits as other people are involved and may depend on your work and decisions as to whether the task is accomplished in a satisfactory way. High-achievement-orientated individuals who are characterised by 'over-commitment' (Siegrist, 1996) may force themselves close to or beyond their ambitions in order to be competitive, to please others and to receive accolades from colleagues and managers on which their self-esteem may depend. It may also be necessary to do one's utmost in order to stay in business. It is always possible to do a little bit more and a little bit better. It is also important for the individual to improve and demonstrate his or her competence in order to be 'employable' rather than 'employed'. As work tasks and work conditions change rapidly over time, the individual's skills and resources determine his or her position in the labour market rather than whether they are in permanent employment. New and changing rules and conditions mean that this type of work situation is expected to increase compared with earlier generations, where workers with a specific manual training, education or skill could expect lifelong employment within stable work context.

The number of low-regulated and boundaryless jobs has increased (Allvin *et al.*, 2011). Regulation in terms of time schedules (nine-to-five, five days a week), a specific workplace where the job is performed and specific regulations regarding what should be done, with whom and under which authority have been replaced by flexibility in terms of time, space and organisation of work. Allvin *et al.* (2011) investigated the amount of flexibility in a randomly selected sample of 4000 individuals representing the working population in Sweden in the age range 23–65 in four aspects: working time, working space, and horizontal and vertical organisation of work. Working time and space were defined by the worker's possibilities for deciding when (during the day, week or year) and where (at the workplace, at home or at other places) he or she is able to perform the job. Horizontal organisation concerns the discretionary power of the worker over the planning of the work, i.e. similar to the 'job decision latitude' dimension of the Karasek (1979) Demand–Control model (see Chapter 4). The vertical dimension of the organisation of work concerns the powers left to the worker to choose informers and collaborators for a specific task or assignment. The results from this study showed that only 16% of Swedish workers are working under traditional conditions regulated in all four aspects, whereas 8% are working under conditions unregulated in all four dimensions. This means that 84% of all workers report that their work is unregulated in at least one of the following dimensions: time, space and horizontal and vertical organisation. Men were found to have unregulated jobs to a larger extent than women. For example, 11% of men had jobs unregulated in all four dimensions compared with only 5% among women.

Telework has made it possible for some employees to choose between working at the office and working from home. This also creates different conditions for those who can and those who cannot use this option owing to the nature of their work tasks or their family situation. Employees serving customers (shop assistants, cashiers in the supermarket, health care personnel) and workers in manual production (assembly workers) have to be at their workplace almost all the time when working. In families with lack of space at home and small children, it may also not be possible to perform telework. For these groups, flexibility in terms of working from home is not an option to reduce stress.

When a governmental agency in Sweden moved their premises from Stockholm to a small nearby city, most employees were offered the possibility of working from home up to three days a week in order to encourage them to stay in the organisation and reduce the time spent on commuting between their home in Stockholm and their new workplace. A study was performed in order to follow up the consequences for the employees (Hanson, 2004). The results show that it was more common for work to interfere with family life than the opposite. The diffuse distinction between work and family life among teleworkers made it unclear when they should stop working, and in order to compensate for this ambiguity most people worked more than necessary. Workers with a higher education usually found it easier to decide when they had done enough and could stop working.

Men and women were also compared in terms of type tasks and stress responses when they were working at the office and when they were working from home. It was found that blood pressure was significantly higher at the office compared with working at home (Lundberg & Lindfors, 2002). One explanation for this difference could be that 'work from home' was made under more peaceful, quiet and undisturbed conditions, and that the work tasks differed. When teleworking at home, people tended to focus on reading and writing reports, planning meetings and problem solving. In the workplace it was more common to interact with other people, and to participate in meetings. In general, this form of flexibility was perceived positively.

It has also been found that telework can induce a greater workload for people who have to stay at the office and undergo the daily chores and to some extent serve those who are working from home or other places. Workers who remain at the office often have to provide information only available at the office, and establish contacts with colleagues within or outside the organisation. Emails and telephone calls from teleworking colleagues requesting rapid information disrupt and interfere with their own work, and create a more stressful work situation. Stress responses such as increased arousal reflected in elevated blood pressure and stress hormone levels affect the quality of performance. For example, creative work, reflection, long-term planning and problem solving are work tasks that are performed more efficiently when the internal arousal level is low, whereas more simple routine tasks (data entry, simple assembly work, answering the telephone in call centres, etc.) can also be performed efficiently at a high arousal level. Workers with intensive demands but limited possibilities for influencing their work situation, for example by teleworking, may thus be less able to perform creative and inventive work and to carry out long-term planning. Thus, it seems as if the employees at this Swedish agency, who were able to choose between work at the office and telework, selected the workplace most suitable for the tasks that they were going to do. It was also found that men working at home had higher adrenaline levels in the evening compared with the levels after working at the office (Lundberg & Lindfors, 2002). This indicates that they were better able to unwind and relax after working at the office, and/or that they continued to work in the evening when working at home.

DIFFUSE DISTINCTION BETWEEN WORK AND OTHER PARTS OF LIFE (FIG. 3.1)

When work can be performed at almost any time and in any place, there is no clear distinction between work and other parts of life such as family, leisure, recreation and sleep. The so-called work–life balance is disturbed (Riedman *et al.*, 2006). 'Flexible work' is usually considered positive and health promoting and there are many advantages with work

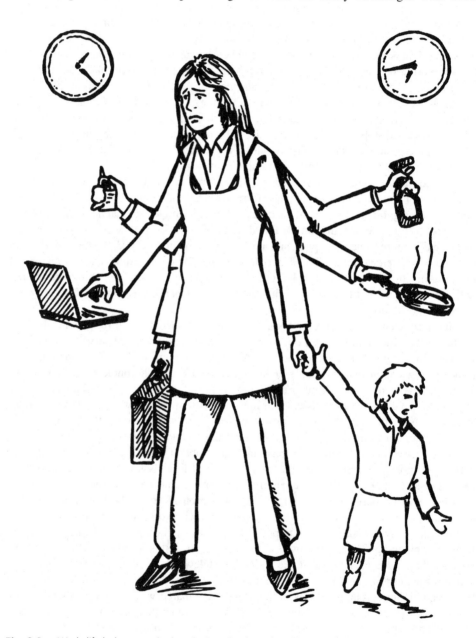

Fig. 3.1   Work–life balance or dual work. Drawing by Urban Skytt.

conditions which are flexible in terms of space and time as long as the worker can decide 'how' to meet the combined loads of work and family responsibilities. Flexibility for the employer, on the other hand, could mean that the worker has to work extra hours and adjust to unforeseen changes and demands in the organisation. This is likely to cause stress, particularly in working parents who depend on predictable working time schedules to meet the needs of their children's timetables, for example at school.

Flexibility for the employee could make it possible to stay at home when feeling ill, or when having to take care of a sick child and still keep in contact with colleagues and perform some work at a distance. With flexible work schedules one can also adjust work according to other more immediate needs, for example putting off important work tasks to the evening when children are asleep or to a weekend day if necessary. The consequences of being away from the workplace for whatever reason may be less serious and can be compensated for. Although this also means an extra burden, it is usually no great problem in the short term but may rather be a relief compared with not being able to perform one's work tasks at all. The possibility of flexibility is not, however, evenly distributed among workers. Managers and people in professional occupations, who are more often men than women, are more likely to have flexible working schedules.

Although flexible work conditions have many advantages, there are also risks involved. Not being able to separate work from other important parts of life and being accessible all the time mean constant activation and reduce the time for rest and recovery. Sleep may be disturbed and reduced because of thoughts about work and apprehension about future demands. Emails, telephone calls and SMS messages may be dropping in around the clock. With more international collaboration, contacts with colleagues living in different time zones sometimes make it necessary to have telephone conferences and other forms of direct communication outside regular working hours. In the long term, this extra burden may contribute to allostatic load (see Chapter 5) and possible health problems. For example, Cohen *et al.* (2009) have recently shown that reduced and disturbed sleep is associated with significantly increased risk of upper respiratory infection. Canivet and colleagues (2008) have demonstrated a prospective relation between sleep problems and increased risk of musculoskeletal disorders. A reasonable balance between activity and rest/recovery is necessary for long-term health (see Chapters 6–8).

A positive consequence of allowing the worker more flexibility is that it encourages more women to enter the labour force and helps people to spend quality time with partner and children. With an increasingly ageing population in Europe, women's participation in the labour force becomes more and more important not only for their own sake but also for society as a whole. Women's participation in the labour market is increasing in all countries, and more flexible work conditions, and working time schedules in particular, are likely to contribute to this trend.

THE CHALLENGE FOR HEALTH AND WELL-BEING IN ORGANISATIONS IN THE FUTURE

In most developed counties, the 1980s and 1990s were described as the decades of the 'enterprise culture', with people working longer and harder to achieve individual success and material rewards. We had globalisation, privatisation, process re-engineering, mergers and acquisitions, strategic alliances, joint ventures and the like, transforming workplaces into hot-house, free-market environments. In the short term this entrepreneurial period improved economic competitiveness in international markets in the countries that embraced it. But as strains began to appear the concept of 'burnout' joined 'junk bonds', 'social networks', and 'outsourcing' in the modern business vocabulary. Nevertheless, work was carried out in essentially the same way as before; it was still business as usual in large or growing medium-sized organisations in US Inc., UK plc, Germany GmBH and so on. By the first decade of the new millennium, a major restructuring of work such as we have never seen since the Industrial Revolution was beginning to take place. The effects of recession and efforts to get out of it have dominated in recent years. Organisations throughout the western world have dramatically downsized, delayered and restructured, and are continuing to do so, in order to keep their labour costs minimal. Whatever euphemism you care to use, the hard reality experienced by many was year-on-year redundancy, constant restructuring and substantial organisational change. Now many organisations are smaller, with fewer people doing more and feeling much less secure. New technology, rather than being our saviour, has added the burden of information overload as well as accelerating the pace of work as a greater speed of response (e.g. smartphones, e-mails) becomes the standard business expectation. At the same time, as more and more companies adopt a global perspective, organisations and the individuals they employ understand that success in the global arena requires fundamental changes in their corporate structures as well as individual competencies. Just as organisations are re-engineering themselves to be more flexible and adaptive, individuals are expected to be open to continual change and life-long learning. Workers will be expected to diagnose their abilities, know where to get appropriate training in deficient skills, know how to network and how to be able to market themselves to organisations professionally, and how to tolerate ambiguity and insecurity (Weinberg & Cooper, 2007).

A FLEXIBLE WORKFORCE

As more organisations outsource, market-test (in the case of the public sector), utilise interim management and the like, many more of us will be selling our services to organisations on a freelance or short-term contract basis. We are creating a corporate culture of blue-collar, white-collar, managerial and professional 'temps': a 'contingent workforce'. In the UK, for example, more than one in ten workers are self-employed; part-time work and the perception of people that they are in effect on short-term contracts are growing faster than permanent full-time work. The number of men in part-time jobs has doubled in the past decade, while the number of people employed by firms of more than 500 employees has slumped to just over one-third of the employed population.

In predicting the look of future corporate life, many experts agree that most organisations will have only a small core of full-time, permanent employees working from a conventional office. They will buy most of the skills they need on a contract basis, either from individuals working at home and linked to the company by computers and other technologies (tele-working), or by hiring people on short-term contracts to do specific jobs or to carry out specific projects. In this way companies will be able to maintain the flexibility they need to cope with a rapidly changing world (Cooper & Jackson, 1997; Sparrow & Cooper, 2003).

This has led to what employers refer to euphemistically as 'the flexible workforce', although in family-friendly terms it is anything but flexible. The 'psychological contract' between employer and employee in terms of 'reasonably permanent employment for work well done' is truly being undermined as more and more employees no longer regard their employment as secure and many more are engaged in part-time work. Indeed, in an ISR (2000) survey of 400 companies in 17 countries employing over 8 million workers throughout Europe, the employment security of workers significantly declined through the mid 1980s to the end of the 1990s: UK, from 70% to 48%; Germany, from 83% to 55%; France, from 64% to 50%; The Netherlands, from 73% to 61%; Belgium, from 60% to 54%; and Italy from 62% to 57%.

It could be argued that there is nothing inherently wrong with this trend, but recent Quality of Working Life Surveys by the Chartered Management Institute (CMI) in the UK (which surveyed a cohort of 10 000 British managers) found some disturbing results (Worrall & Cooper, 2001, 2007). It was found that over 60% of this national sample of managers had undergone major restructuring over the last 12 months, involving major downsizing and outsourcing. The consequences of this change, even among an occupational group (i.e. middle and senior managers) supposedly in control of events, were that nearly two out of three experienced increased job insecurity, lowered morale, and the erosion of motivation and loyalty.

Most of these changes involved downsizing, cost reduction, delayering and outsourcing. Yet the perception was that although inevitably these changes led to an increase in profitablity and productivity, decision-making was slower and, more importantly, the organisation was deemed to have lost the right mix of human resource skills and experience in the process.

In addition, the impact on working patterns was penal, both from a business point of view and in terms of managers' outside lives. This was partly due not only to more work being imposed on the metaphorical 'backs of fewer managers', but also to 'presenteeism', the need for managers to demonstrate commitment by working longer and unsocial hours – behaviour which they felt (possibly falsely) would protect them from the next wave of redundancies.

In the most recent survey (Worrall & Cooper, 2007), it was found that 89% of executives regularly work over their contracted hours, with nearly 40% working at least two hours more per day. In addition, whereas a third of this cohort of executives in 1997 felt that their employer expected them to put in these hours, by 2001 this had risen to nearly 60%. What is also disturbing about this trend towards a long-hours culture is the managers' perception of the damage it is inflicting on them and their families: 94% of these executives reported that these hours damaged their health, 63% that it adversely affected their relationship with their children, 59% that it damaged their relationship with their partner, and 60% that long hours reduced their productivity.

This trend towards a long-hours culture and intrinsic job insecurity was also having an effect on the family as more and more two-earner families/couples emerged in a climate that was anything but 'family friendly' (Swann & Cooper, 2005).

Consequences of changing employment relationships

So what are the consequences of the changing nature of the psychological contract between employer and employee? Sparrow & Cooper (2003) identified four areas that are affected by changing employment relationships at work:

1. What we want out of work and how we maintain individuality in a world where we face a choice between more intense employment or no employment at all.
2. Our relationships with other individuals in a work process that can be altered in terms of social interactions, time patterns and geographical locations.

3. The co-operative and competitive links between different internal and external consti-
   tuents of the organisation in their new more flexible forms.
4. The relationships between key stakeholders and institutions such as governments, unions
   and managers.

In addition to changing relationships at work, there are a number of consequences of
the way we work. First, as more and more people work from their home, whether part-time
or on a short-term contract, we will be increasingly creating 'virtual organisations'. The big
corporate question here is: how will the 'virtual organisation' of the future manage this
dispersed workforce when communication difficulties are already apparent in existing
structures (Worrall & Cooper, 2007).

Second, with two out of three families/couples two-earner or dual career, how will working
from home affect the delicate balance between home and work, or indeed the division of roles
between men and women? Indeed, with employers increasingly looking for and recruiting
'flexible workers', will not women be preferred to men given their history of flexibility? For
example, in the UK, there are currently five times as many women working part-time as men.
Although twice as many men are now working part-time than a decade ago, women are
historically more experienced at discontinuous career patterns, flowing in and out of the
labour market, working part-time and on short-term contracts (Lewis & Cooper, 2005).

Third, since the Industrial Revolution, many white-collar, managerial and professional
workers have not experienced high levels of job insecurity. Even many blue-collar workers
who were laid off in the heavy manufacturing industries of the past were frequently re-
employed when times got better. The question that society has to ask itself is: Can human
beings cope with permanent job insecurity without the safety and security of organisational
structures which in the past provided training, development and careers? The European
survey by ISR (1995) provided some cause for concern in this regard, showing the UK with
the worst decline in employee satisfaction in terms of employment insecurity of any of its
competitors, from 70% satisfaction levels in 1985 to 47% by 1995 to 2000; at a time when UK
plc has been moving faster towards a contingent workforce than any of its European
counterparts – a fate soon to be felt by other Europeans.

Will this trend towards stable insecurity, freelance working and virtual organisations
continue? And, more importantly, can organisations, virtual or otherwise, continue to
demand commitment from employees to whom they do not commit? In comparative terms
the UK economy is doing remarkably well, but levels of job insecurity and dissatisfaction are
fairly high. Developing and maintaining a 'feelgood' factor at work and in our economy
generally is not just about bottom-line factors (e.g. higher salaries, lowering of income tax, or
increased profitability). It is, or should be in a civilised society, about quality-of-life issues as
well, such as hours of work, family time, manageable workloads, control over one's career
and some sense of job security. As the social anthropologist Studs Terkel (1972) suggested,
'Work is about a search for daily meaning as well as daily bread, for recognition as well as
cash, for astonishment rather than torpor, in short, for a sort of life rather than a Monday
through Friday sort of dying'.

Spector et al. (2007) compared work demands, job satisfaction and turnover intentions
with work–family conflict among managers in four clusters of countries, one with a
collectivistic culture (Asia, East Europe and Latin America) and one with a more individ-
ualist orientation (Anglo). In countries with an individualistic culture, individuals are
focusing more on their own needs, whereas people in collectivistic countries view themselves
in terms of social relations to co-workers and their employer and are willing to sacrifice their

own needs in favour of the larger collective. In all, 5270 managers from 20 countries participated in the study. In general, a stronger association between work demand and work–family conflict was seen in individualistic countries, such as West European countries and the USA, compared with more collectivistic countries in Asia and Latin America. It was also found that perceived workload was more important than working hours. Job satisfaction and turnover intentions of people in individualistic countries were more affected by work interfering with family life compared with people in collectivistic countries. Possible explanations for these findings are that people in collectivistic countries have greater availability of domestic support from society as well as from extended family and friends and from paid domestic help and/or that women in Asia and Latin America do not have a paid job as often as women in Europe and North America.

The role of gender

One target of the European Foundation for the Improvement of Living and Working Conditions (2009) policy is to raise the employment rate among women, particularly those older than 55 years. In addition to the gender perspective, one important reason is the demographic changes in Europe, with a growing elderly population. According to statistics, older women (55–64 years) represent an increasing proportion of the workforce in the EU, but there are great differences between countries. Whereas there is almost no difference in employment rate between men and women in the Nordic countries, there is a gender difference of about 20% in Cyprus, Greece, Ireland, Italy and Spain and a 40% difference in Malta. One important reason for these differences between countries is access to childcare facilities and their cost. In Sweden, for instance, every family is offered high-quality childcare from the local community at a low cost as this service is mainly financed via general taxation. Access to informal childcare often provided by grandparents has also decreased as grandparents are still in employment or too old to take care of children because they had their first child rather late in life. However, in general, female participation in the workforce has grown for several reasons. Women have a desire for an occupational career and an independent income, and more flexible working practices have made it easier to combine work and family responsibilities. An income is usually also necessary for maternity benefits and for a reasonable pension in old age.

Older women workers and women with small children more often work part time, and a higher proportion of them are on temporary and insecure contracts compared with men of the same age. In Britain, for instance, there are currently five times as many women as men working part-time. Women are still concentrated in certain occupational groups, such as care workers, clerical staff and service and sales workers, and are paid less than men. Women spend more time than men in unpaid domestic work (childcare, household duties, etc.), and it has been found that women working part time have a greater total workload than men working full time.

The labour market for men is more differentiated than it is for women. Twenty seven per cent of all Swedish women work within the five most common women's occupations, that is, nursing assistants, licensed nurses, preschool teachers and recreation leaders, childminders and office staff. Only 15% of all men work within the five most common men's occupations: company sales representatives, mechanical engineers and technicians, data specialists, warehouse and shipping assistants, and truck drivers. More women than men work with people in emotionally demanding jobs, which is likely to be an extra burden and will further reduce their opportunities for rest and recovery.

Lundberg *et al.* (1994) and Berntsson *et al.* (2005) compared full-time employed male and female Swedish white-collar workers matched for age, occupation and family situation with regard to paid and unpaid workload and responsibility for home and family. Even among highly educated full-time employed men and women, for example male and female physicians, psychologists, chemists and administrators, women with children consistently reported a greater total workload than did men, and the gender difference increased with the number of children. In families with three children or more, the gender difference in total workload was about 18 hours per week (Lundberg *et al.*, 1994). In addition, women were more often found to carry the main responsibility for all items related to childcare (caring for infants, taking children to and from school, helping with school work, etc.) and almost all types of household chores (shopping, cooking, cleaning, ironing, washing up, etc.) except regular maintenance and repair of the house/apartment and the car, and managing finances (Fig. 3.2). Similar gender differences have been found in several other countries (e.g. Kahn, 1991; Gjerdingen *et al.*, 2000).

Despite equal opportunity legislation and encouragement of women to have professional careers, there are still considerably fewer women than men in managerial positions. Where women do occupy managerial positions, this tends to be in the health and education sectors, and women occupy lower hierarchical positions than do male managers. There are different reasons for this. Active discrimination cannot be excluded, but more indirect reasons could be the prevalence of a male model of work, where 'male' competence is considered more valuable than 'female' competence. Managers are expected to work continuously from the end of education to retirement without breaks for childbirth, and to work long hours and not allow family matters to interfere with work. Women in dual-career families are still carrying out the main responsibility for domestic duties, so those who take managerial responsibility may end up with an extremely heavy total workload (paid plus unpaid work). This is likely to make women more reluctant to take additional managerial responsibility, which would cause a further increase in workload.

The negative consequences of the conflict between work and family life are also likely to contribute to the dramatic decline in birth rate in Europe, and in southern Europe in particular. Young workers decide not to have children in order to focus entirely on their occupational career and personal development. In the near future, this will cause an imbalance between age groups and a large proportion of elderly people to be supported and cared for by a decreasing number of young people. To some extent this trend can be compensated for by increased immigration of young people from other parts of the world where the population structure in terms of age is quite different with a large part of the population aged 20 or younger (discussed further below). Immigration is, however, likely to have only a moderate influence on future demographic structure in Europe.

None the less, there is potential for change in women's occupational opportunities. Economic incentives and a personal interest in developing an occupational career, more flexible working arrangements and national and international policies promoting equal opportunities for women and men, are expected to contribute to decrease the differences between men's and women's occupational conditions. Today in many countries girls are doing better than boys at school and are thus more competitive for places in higher education. More highly educated women compared with men would make them more attractive on the labour market. There is also evidence that women leaders tend to be more open, approachable and encouraging to others (Rosener, 1990; Gibson, 1995) and able to create an atmosphere of participative safety in teams. In rapidly changing workplaces these competencies are likely to become more and more important.

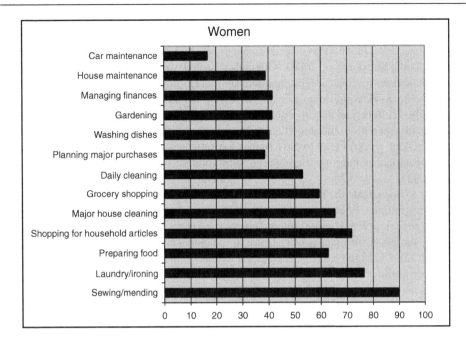

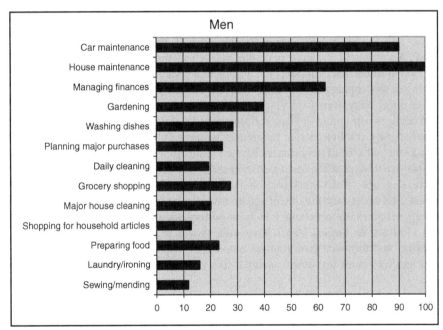

Fig. 3.2 Proportion of women and men, respectively (%), taking the main responsibility for household duties. Reprinted from Berntsson *et al.* (2005) with permission.

The role of age and tenure

The negative effects of job stress on performance seem to decrease with years of employment (Sturman, 2003; Shirom *et al.*, 2008). Although a 'healthy worker effect' cannot be excluded, likely explanations for this moderating effect are that employees who stay at their jobs adapt to the specific work conditions, gain knowledge and increase their understanding of the organisational culture, and thereby enhance their ability to cope with job stressors. As people age they gain experience, allowing them to become more effective in the use of their coping resources. Older workers tend to have higher job satisfaction, job involvement, motivation and organisational commitment compared with younger workers (Cohen & Wills, 1985; Cohen, 1993).

In order to investigate the moderators of the relationships between work-related stressors and job performance, Fried and colleagues (2008) focused on three demographic variables, employee gender, age and tenure, and the influence of stressors such as role conflict and role ambiguity on job performance. Data from 30 independent studies with 7700 participants were used. Role ambiguity was defined as the extent to which employees are unclear about their responsibilities, or when role-related expectations are unclear. 'Role conflict' was defined as the extent to which employees experience conflicting demands at work. Tenure and gender were not found to moderate the effects of stress on performance, but increasing employee mean age had a moderating effect on the role ambiguity–performance relationship. The reduction in the negative relationship between role ambiguity and performance with increasing age and tenure was more pronounced in female- than in male-dominated workplaces.

Taylor (2006) has described a specific female mode of coping with stress, called 'tend-and-befriend'. According to this mode of coping, women are more likely to form social networks and support systems that counteract the detrimental effects of stress. It seems reasonable to conclude that this coping resource increases with age and years of employment and thus has a positive effect on performance. Another factor contributing to the decline in the negative relation between role ambiguity and performance in women is that older women experience less work–family conflict relative to younger women. Differences in men's and women's work tasks may also be of importance. Women more often tend to work with people (e.g. in caring jobs, teaching positions) and men more often with things (e.g. in manufacturing). With the increasing age of the workforce in many countries, it becomes more important to investigate and understand the role of age in stress and performance. A positive effect of age on coping resources has beneficial effects on performance under stressful work conditions. Studies (Rhodes & Steers, 1990) have also shown that older employees have lower absenteeism and turnover than younger employees. However, in jobs requiring physical exertion and very quick responses, ageing is likely to have negative effects on performance.

4 Work as a Source of Stimulation and Health or a Cause of Distress and Illness

WORK-RELATED STRESS MODELS

A number of models have been proposed in order to describe the factors that link work with stress-related disorders, and those that enable work to contribute to stimulation, well-being and health (Karasek & Theorell, 1990; Lundberg, 2007; Richter *et al.*, 2007; Schnall *et al.*, 2009). Frankenhaeuser (1986) and others have emphasised the importance of a reasonable balance between perceived work demands and the individual's perceived own resources to meet these demands. Karasek (1979) and Karasek and Theorell (1990) have formulated a model based on the relation between work demands and the possibilities for influence and control. In addition to the two original dimensions, social support has been included as a third dimension of this model (Johnson & Hall, 1988). A third model used to measure stress at work in many recent studies is the Effort–Reward–Imbalance model of Siegrist (1996). More recently, Ursin and Eriksen (2004) have formulated the Cognitive Activation Theory of Stress (CATS). CATS is based on formal logistic definitions of stress concepts, and can be applied to all forms of stress in humans and animals in order to predict positive and negative health outcomes.

When the individual's perceived resources are in balance with the perceived demands, the work situation is considered to be stimulating and pleasant (Fig. 4.1). This model of work-related stress is based on the individual's perceptions, which means that imbalance and stress could be induced because an individual underestimates his or her actual resources or overestimates the anticipated demands. Low self-esteem is likely to increase the risk that even moderate work demands will induce stress in certain individuals. It is easy to see that stress will occur when the demands exceed the individual's resources, which happens when the worker is facing quantitatively or qualitatively overwhelming work tasks, conflicts between demands and/or extremely long working hours. These can be described as different forms of overstimulation. However, according to this model, imbalance between demands and resources may also be caused by the opposite situation: the demands are too low compared with the worker's resources: a form of understimulation. Not being able to use one's experiences, education, training, skills and abilities also induces stress. Understimulation is likely to occur in simple repetitive assembly work, in data entry and certain forms of

The Science of Occupational Health: Stress, Psychobiology and the New World of Work, first edition
By Ulf Lundberg and Cary L. Cooper. Published 2011 by Blackwell Publishing Ltd
© 2011 Ulf Lundberg and Cary L. Cooper

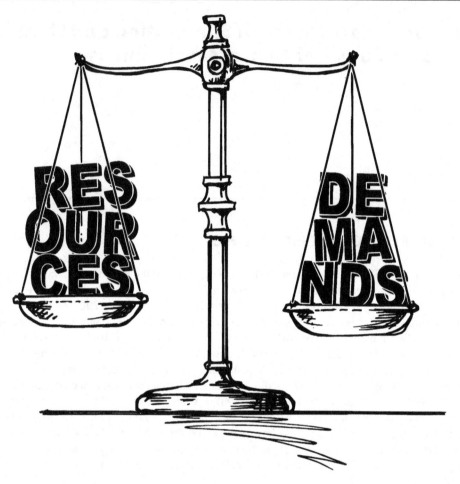

Fig. 4.1 Balance between demands and resources promotes health, well-being and performance. Drawing by Urban Skytt.

surveillance jobs (Lundberg & Johansson, 2000), but also in situations characterised by lack of meaningful activities, such as among unemployed people, people on sick leave and after retirement from work. Understimulation may also exist among highly educated immigrants who have to take very simple jobs because they cannot speak the language in their new homeland well enough, have the 'wrong' education or are subjected to discrimination. This kind of stress due to understimulation may explain the fact that unemployment is often associated with mental and physical health problems (Grossi, 2008). Intuitively, it seems paradoxical that individuals without any work demands at all are under stress, but experimental studies show that understimulation induces stress responses and symptoms similar to what happens during overstimulation (Frankenhaeuser, 1971). Britton and Shipley (2010) investigated the relation between boredom (not at all, a little, quite a lot, all the time) and health outcomes, including lifestyle, in 7524 men and women from the Whitehall II study. Mortality, especially from CHD, was significantly higher among those with a great deal of boredom compared with those not bored at all. The study indicated that boredom could be

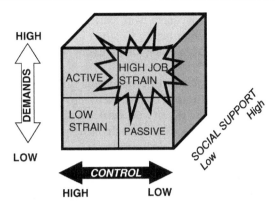

Fig. 4.2   The Demand–Control–Support model.

related to CHD risk factors such as excessive drinking, smoking, taking drugs and poor self-rated health.

The Demand–Control–Support model has resulted in the Job Content Questionnaire (Theorell, 2008), which has been translated into a number of different languages and used extensively in work, stress and health research (Fig. 4.2). The Demand–Control–Support model has similarities to the Demand–Resources–Balance model, and was initially based on the combinations of two dimensions, 'demand' and 'control'. *Job demands* refer to mental and/or physical work demands, high work pace, etc., and are defined by questions such as 'working very fast', 'working very hard', and 'not enough time to get the job done'. *Control* refers to actual control over the work situation in terms of pace and work tasks but also job decision latitude, that is, the individual's ability to influence methods and routines, the decision-making authority available to the worker, and opportunities to take responsibility and to be able to use his/her skill and ability. By combining the dimensions of demand and control, four different work situations can be identified. The combination of high demands and high levels of control represents an active work situation, considered to induce stimulation, motivation, high job satisfaction, well-being, health and high productivity. Workers considered to belong to this category include scientists, managing directors and chief executive officers of organisations and companies. High social support at work will further contribute to induce high job satisfaction and additional positive emotions. Social support at work comprises good relations with co-workers and management, help when needed, and feedback. High demands combined with low levels of control represent high job strain, a stress-related work situation causing low job satisfaction, distress and health problems. A waiter in a restaurant, a cashier at the supermarket and an assembly line worker could serve as examples of jobs in this category. Combined with lack of social support the worker's vulnerability in high-strain jobs will increase even more. Considerable evidence exists that link 'job strain' to hypertension, CHD and other disorders (Kivimäki *et al.*, 2006; Theorell, 2008).

The other two combinations, 'low work demands and high job control' and 'low work demands and low job control', respectively, are described as 'low-strain work' and 'passive' work. Low-strain work does not constitute a health problem, whereas 'passive' work may represent a form of understimulation and, hence, be associated with stress responses and symptoms. Social support from colleagues and management is important for health and work satisfaction. Continuous adequate feedback regarding work achievements contributes to greater job involvement and should include both encouragement and appreciation of good achievements and criticism for inadequate work performance. Uncertainty about what is expected from the employer is contributing to stress and insecurity. The possibility of receiving help when needed is also important for increasing work satisfaction and security at work and reduces stress.

Research on effort–reward imbalance (ERI) and health is focused on the notion of 'social reciprocity'. Taking a job means a form of contract between the employer and the employee. The employer expects the employee to carry out certain tasks, and the employee expects to receive an adequate reward for doing so. The reward is usually in terms of economic payment, but can also consist of or be combined with good career opportunities, high job security, status and appreciation (Siegrist, 1996). Failed reciprocity elicits effort–reward imbalance and strong negative emotions associated with sustained stress responses. Appropriate social rewards evoke positive emotions and promote well-being and health. High effort, combined with low reward at work, is particularly deleterious for individuals characterised by excessive work-related commitment, who find it difficult or impossible to stop thinking about work (who show 'overcommitment'). The ERI model has been very successful in predicting stress-related health problems at work, and has a potential also to be relevant for predicting health in a rapidly changing work environment (Siegrist, 2008).

Ursin and Eriksen (2004) have created a formal system of definitions of stress concepts based on expectations of success or failure, the Cognitive Activation Theory of Stress (CATS), which is relevant for stress responses in all species. According to this model, anticipation of success, e.g. 'I know that I can handle the situation', 'I will manage', activates the individual by increasing mental and physiological arousal but is not associated with harmful effects. A moderate increase in arousal is followed by a rapid return to baseline (rest) when the challenge is over. However, perceiving that 'Things are out of my control', 'The outcome depends on chance, on other people, on fate, etc,' will induce feelings of helplessness and is associated with prolonged stress responses and increased risk of mental and physical disorders. Catastrophic thoughts such as expecting that 'Whatever I do in this situation, I will fail' will induce feelings of 'hopelessness' and chronic stress activation and, eventually distress, anxiety, depression and a number of stress-related disorders as described in Chapter 6. The discrepancy between what is expected and the individual's perceived coping resources determines the magnitude of the stress response. Short-term activation does not constitute a threat to health, but if sustained the response may lead to illness and disease through established pathophysiological processes ('allostatic load'). An important contribution of the CATS model is that it defines some rather vague stress-related concepts in terms of clear formal logical expressions, and is relevant for distinguishing between stressful conditions that are harmless and harmful in both humans and animals. Animals repeatedly exposed to uncontrollable stress in terms of mild electric shocks are known to develop a condition named 'learned helplessness'. For example, dogs that had previously 'learned' that nothing they did had any effect on whether or not they received unpleasant shocks simply lay down passively and did not even try to escape when exposed to new shocks (Seligman, 1975).

Phenomena similar to 'learned helplessness' also exist among humans who have repeatedly been exposed to 'uncontrollable stress'. People who feel that, whatever they do, their lives are determined by chance, fate, environmental conditions or other people are at risk of developing depression and give up attempts to change their lives even when it is possible. This is related to the concept of 'locus of control' (Rotter, 1966), where 'external locus of control' is similar to learned helplessness, whereas 'internal locus of control' represents a belief that the individual to a large extent can determine and control his or her own life. Internal locus of control and a similar concept by Antonovsky (1987), 'sense of coherence', are examples of individual 'salutogenetic' factors counteracting the negative effects of stress (more on this in Chapter 10).

The different work-related stress models described above have similarities, and the concepts overlap to some extent. In general, high work stress defined according to all these models is related to negative health outcomes, but results are not quite consistent. The models are not identical but represent slightly different aspects of work-related stress, and some models are more relevant than others depending on the type of work situation. The Demand–Control or job strain model was mainly developed on the basis of industrial work, whereas the ERI and the CATS models are relevant also for 'knowledge intensive' and service sectors. In conclusion, these models are complementary rather than competitive. For example, Ostry *et al.* (2003) compared the predictive validity of the job strain and ERI models, alone and in combination with each other, for self-reported health status and the self-reported presence of any chronic disease condition. They found that the two models independently predicted poor self-reported health status. The ERI model, but not the job strain model, also predicted the presence of a chronic disease. A model combining 'effort–reward imbalance' and 'task-level control' was found to be a better predictor of self-reported health status and chronic disease than either model alone.

JUSTICE

'Justice' is also important for health and well-being at work. Kivimäki, Ferrie *et al.* (2005) examined 'justice at work' as a predictor of CHD in a prospective study of 6442 male British civil servants (Whitehall II) aged 35 to 55 years without prevalent CHD at baseline. Perceived justice at work was determined by means of questionnaire, and incidence of CHD was based on medical records during a 9-year follow-up. After controlling for age, employment grade and traditional risk factors for CHD, such as baseline cholesterol concentration, body mass index, hypertension, smoking, alcohol consumption and physical activity, employees who experienced a high level of justice at work had a lower risk of CHD than employees with a low or intermediate level of justice. The level of justice remained an independent predictor of CHD also after adjustment for job strain and effort–reward imbalance.

Semmer *et al.* (2010) have recently described a new source of stress at work named 'illegitimate tasks', which refers to the request to employees to perform unreasonable or unnecessary work tasks or tasks that are incompatible with one's occupational status. For example, it is unreasonable to ask a medical doctor at a hospital to serve as a receptionist or ask an electrician to do cleaning work. These tasks are outside the range of tasks reasonably expected from persons with these occupations. Asking a person to do meaningless or completely unnecessary tasks, such as manually typing in text that could easily be scanned electronically is also a form of violation of the norms and offends the worker. Semmer *et al.* (2010) admit that the concept of 'illegitimate tasks' to some extent overlaps that of 'role conflict' but is more specific: 'any type of task may be illegitimate in a specific situation for a specific person' (p. 75).

POSITIVE AND NEGATIVE WORK (FIG. 4.3)

Work is important for many reasons. It gives life a time structure and contributes to meaning, status, variation, social relationships and personal development and, of course, to necessary

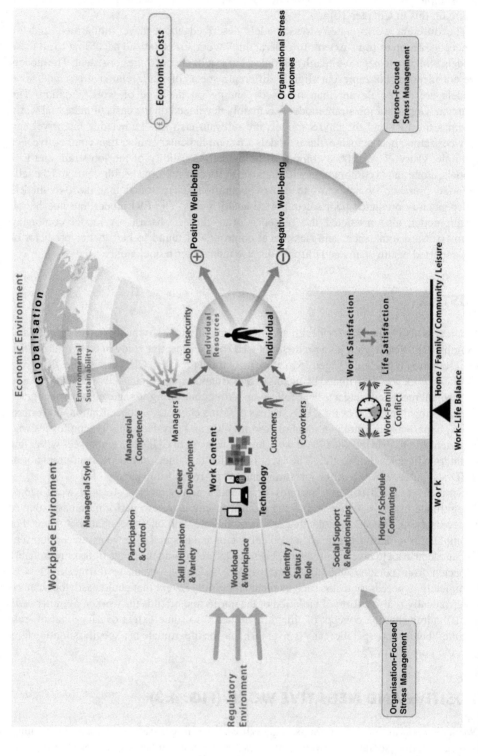

Fig. 4.3 An overview of the key factors that influence well-being at work. (Source: Foresight Mental Capital & Well-Being Project 2008.)

economic resources. Research consistently shows that women employed outside the home have better mental and physical health and live longer than homemakers, even after controlling for the fact that one has to be healthy to take and hold a job. Next to family and good health, work is often rated as the most important thing in life.

'Negative work' stress is more strongly linked to morbidity than stress induced by high job involvement and work overload due to high commitment and interest. However, positive job involvement is no guarantee against stress-related disorders, as demonstrated by, for example, the *karoshi* phenomenon described below, and research on the Type A behaviour pattern (Friedman & Rosenman, 1959; Rosenman & Chesney, 1980). A difference between the consequences of negative and positive job stress is that negative stress usually has a long-term impact on people with elevated physiological stress levels even when they are off work. If you feel insecure, or when you are dissatisfied with your job, boss or colleagues, it can be difficult to stop thinking about work when something negative has happened. This is likely to induce a high allostatic load (see Chapter 5). A high positive workload in a stimulating and interesting job, on the other hand, makes unwinding outside work easier and quicker. After a successful, pleasant and interesting day at the job, it is natural to feel satisfied and it is easier to unwind and relax. However, if the individual is 'overcommitted' and cannot relax from work in evenings and during weekends and holidays, there will not be enough time for rest and recovery. Consequently, allostatic load will accumulate even if the work in itself is stimulating. Positive work involvement and overtime work are common in jobs that focus on information technology and administration.

Modern work conditions could mean more influence and control for the worker and greater responsibility. Up to a certain level, individual responsibility is health promoting and productive. However, when too much responsibility is put on the individual, especially when combined with diffuse goals and unclear expectations from the employer, this may become a burden rather than a resource. The employee may feel forced to exert extra effort and time in order to meet these unclear demands, which means constant striving and increased allostatic load.

JOB SATISFACTION

Factors known to be of particular importance for job satisfaction and stress levels are the number of hours of work, organisational culture, management style, workload and autonomy/control. A number of studies suggest a link between low job satisfaction and ill health. Job satisfaction is determined on the basis of the employee's feelings of having an interesting job, good relationships with colleagues and managers, good career opportunities, independent work and an adequate income. Faragher *et al.* (2005) performed a systematic review and meta-analysis of 485 studies with a total sample size of 267995 individuals in order to evaluate the role of job satisfaction for physical and mental well-being. It was found that low job satisfaction was strongly linked to burnout, depression and anxiety and modestly related to subjective physical illness. By identifying the most important risk factors for dissatisfaction among employees, health intervention programmes can be designed.

Harter *et al.* (2002) investigated nearly 8000 separate business units in 36 companies and found that 'engagement and well-being' were linked to business unit performance in terms of such factors as customer satisfaction, productivity, profitability, employee turnover and sickness absence. The meta-analysis (Harter *et al.*, 2002) indicated a stronger relation between job satisfaction and job performance than was previously evident. A general assumption is that happy workers are more productive. Hosie *et al.* (2007) investigated whether Australian managers' job-related affective well-being and job satisfaction were related to their performance. They measured affective well-being with two established scales covering (1) negative affect (distressed, upset, etc.) and positive affect (interested, excited, etc.), and (2) enthusiasm, anxiety, depression, relaxation and job satisfaction (amount of variety, recognition for good work, opportunity to use your abilities, promotion opportunities, attention, responsibility and freedom). Managers' contextual performance was measured by means of a scale with four factors: endorsing (concern, loyalty, etc.), helping (helping others, etc.), persisting (perseverance, extra effort, etc.) and following (obeying rules, adherence, care, etc.). Managers' task performance was measured by self-ratings covering the following four factors: monitoring (controlling, etc.), technical (solving technical problems and applying technical expertise, etc.), influencing (inside and outside the organisation, persuading, convincing, etc.), and delegating (assigning staff duties, etc.). It was found that positive affect and enthusiasm had a positive association with all the performance dimensions. Affective well-being and job satisfaction were associated with managers' performance irrespective of whether the performance scores were from self-reports or superiors' ratings. In conclusion, by improving managers' affective well-being and job satisfaction, performance and organisational effectiveness will increase. However, it is also possible that managers' well-being and job satisfaction increase when their performance is effective.

Research on occupational stress and health has consistently shown that lack of influence and control, work overload, conflicting demands and instructions, lack of leadership or bad management and repetitive and monotonous work tasks contribute to stress and stress-related disorders (Karasek & Theorell, 1990; Lundberg & Johansson, 2000; Richter *et al.*, 2007; Schnall *et al.*, 2009). Work-induced stress has also been associated with remaining stress after work (Melin *et al.*, 1999; Lundberg & Johansson, 2000). When stress from work remains after work, opportunities for rest and recovery are reduced. Lack of rest is likely to be at least as important for mental and physical health as mental and physical stress at work itself (see Chapter 5).

WORKAHOLISM

Personality characteristics, partly developed as a consequence of the work climate, such as being a workaholic and being overcommitted, may cause additional stress in the employee. Overcommitment is reflected in a tendency to always strain oneself close to or beyond one's limit in order to please others and receive appreciation. The concept 'workaholic' has been used to describe individuals who are addicted to work and consider it the most or only important thing in life. An extreme form of workaholic may show *karoshi*, a phenomenon that has been noticed in Japan and identified as a serious work-related health outcome. It means that someone is working almost without breaks and rest until he or she dies due to complete exhaustion. The major medical causes of *karoshi* deaths are heart attack (myocardial infarction) and stroke (Chapter 6). This phenomenon is reported in Japanese occupational health statistics, and the number of *karoshi* deaths has increased in recent years. This is assumed to be due to increasing stress from work demands, competition and overcommitment to work among Japanese employees.

Unexpected natural death has also been observed among South Korean workers and has been suggested to be related to occupational stress and overwork. Park *et al.* (1999) investigated epidemiological components and work stress associated with workers' natural deaths in South Korea (812 male and 82 female cases) in comparison with a matched control group. Cerebrovascular disorder, that is, dysfunctions related to the blood vessels supplying the brain, was the most common reason for death, representing 47% of the cases, followed by heart (coronary artery) disease causing 30% of the deaths. It was concluded that unexpected natural death might be influenced by work stress, but that more research is needed to identify the exact mechanisms leading to cerebrovascular and cardiovascular attacks among middle-aged workers.

TYPE A BEHAVIOUR

In the 1970s and 1980s, numerous studies were performed on the Type A or coronary-prone behaviour pattern. Type A behaviour was first described by two cardiologists, Meyer Friedman and Ray Rosenman (1959). They found that many of their cardiac patients expressed certain characteristics, such as impatience, time urgency, competitiveness and job involvement. Interest in this stress-related behaviour pattern increased after two longitudinal studies supporting a causal relationship between Type A behaviour and coronary heart disease (CHD). The Western Collaborative Group Study (Rosenman *et al.*, 1976) comprised about 3000 middle-aged men, who were classified as Type A or Type B (lacking Type A characteristics) on the basis of an interview involving both verbal (actual responses to questions) and non-verbal (mimics, gestures, choice of words, etc.) information (the Structured Interview). These men were followed up for 8.5 years and it was found that the number of heart attacks was about twice as high among Type A individuals compared with their Type B counterparts after controlling for traditional coronary risk factors (high blood pressure, high blood lipids, diabetes, overweight, smoking). Similar results were obtained from the Framingham Heart Study (Haynes *et al.*,1978a, b) based on both women and men. These results were accepted as evidence for a relationship between this behaviour pattern and CHD in addition to and of the same magnitude as previously identified physical risk factors (Weiss, 1981).

Some typical characteristcs of Type A behaviour

- Time urgency: walk fast, talk fast, eat fast, even when there is plenty of time.
- Impatience: get easily irritated when having to queue and having to wait.
- Competitiveness: like to compete and win.
- Job involvement: high work pace, work is the most important thing in life.
- Aggression, hostility: get angry easily, don't trust other people, need to control others.

These findings stimulated research on the possible psychobiological mechanisms involved. Results from a great number of studies showed that Type A individuals responded to relevant challenges, such as competition, lack of control and queueing, with a more pronounced increase in physiological stress responses, for example increased blood pressure, heart rate and stress hormone output compared with Type B individuals. Repeatedly elevated heart rate and blood pressure in response to mental challenges is assumed to contribute to cardiovascular disorders (Chapter 6). In recent decades the interest in Type A behaviour has declined considerably. One reason for this is that more and more people would be classified as Type A individuals today according the original criteria. Increased occupational demands for efficiency, job involvement, time pressure and competitiveness have induced more Type A behaviour in a large part of the population and, consequently, the predictive power of Type A behaviour has been reduced.

At the same time the prevalence of CHD has decreased about 50% in the working population in the USA and Western Europe since 1980. The reason for the reduction in CHD in the working population is probably that medical check-ups are performed more frequently, and medication against high blood pressure and high blood lipids has become more common and the drugs are more efficient. In addition, cigarette smoking has decreased markedly among men in the USA and Western Europe, dietary habits have improved and regular physical exercise is practised in large parts of the population, particularly in high socioeconomic status groups. Furthermore, as large-scale prospective studies are expensive and time consuming, very few studies on Type A behaviour and CHD have been performed in recent years. The longitudinal studies on Type A behaviour and CHD performed in the 1970s and 1980s have, however, shown that a stress-related behaviour pattern can predict a fatal somatic disease such as heart attack (myocardial infarction) independently of other physical risk factors for CHD (Weiss, 1981). Heart attacks were earlier considered to be a managerial disease but are now more common among manual workers (Marmot & Shipley, 1996).

In a longitudinal study Barefoot *et al.* (1983) measured hostility in 255 physicians using the Cook–Medley Hostility Scale, and found a strong association between high hostility scores and cardiovascular events and mortality 25 years later. Individuals with hostility scores above a certain level around the age of 25 were six times as likely to have died after 25 years compared with individuals with scores below that level. This and other studies have focused interest on the role of hostility in heart disease, and Williams *et al.* (1980) have concluded that hostility is the most 'toxic' component of Type A behaviour. Räikkönen *et al.* (2004) followed 290 healthy women and found that trait anger predicted progression of carotid atherosclerosis. Results also suggested that this association was mediated by the metabolic syndrome (see Chapter 6).

The Framingham Heart Study (Haynes *et al.*, 1978a, b) involved both women and men and showed that Type A behaviour could also be a risk factor for women. However, Type A behaviour was defined by Rosenman and Friedman on the basis of male cardiac patients, and it is generally defined by traditional masculine characteristics: aggression, competitiveness, impatience and job involvement. Consequently, most studies on Type A behaviour have been performed on men and therefore the relation between Type A behaviour and CHD in women is unclear. One reason for the focus on men is, of course, that heart attacks are between four and five times as common in middle-aged men compared with middle-aged women. However, heart disease kills more women than men each year but strikes women, on average, 10 years later than men.

JOB STRAIN AND HEART DISORDER

Additional support for a relationship between job stress and CHD comes from a number of studies. For example, Kuper and Marmot (2003) investigated the association between job strain and components of the job strain model and CHD risk in the prospective Whitehall II study with 6895 male and 3413 female civil servants aged 35–55. It was found that job strain, high job demands and, to some extent, low decision latitude, were associated with an increased risk of CHD. Using the Karasek job strain model of psychological demands/

control, Kornitzer *et al.* (2006) investigated six cohorts from four European countries consisting of 21 111 middle-aged male subjects. During a mean follow-up of 40 months, 185 acute coronary events or coronary deaths were observed. The job strain model was found to be an independent predictor of acute coronary events, with the psychological demands scale emerging as the most important component. Netterstrøm *et al.* (2006) performed a prospective study based on the job strain model of 659 employed healthy men as part of the World Health Organization-initiated MONICA II project. Classification of the components in the job strain model was made objectively from job titles and subjectively from questionnaires. All participants were followed for 13 years with regard to hospitalisation and death as a result of ischaemic heart disease (IHD). Self-reported job strain and high demands, but not objective classification of the components in the job strain model, were significantly associated with IHD, independently of standard coronary risk factors.

In a meta-analysis of 14 prospective cohort studies involving 83 014 employees, Kivimäki *et al.* (2006) investigated the association between work stress and CHD. Data suggest that work stress was associated with a 50% excess risk for CHD. Similar findings have been reported by, among others, Hemingway and Marmot (1999) and Belkic *et al.* (2004). In a review of a number of risk factors for myocardial infarction, involving 15 152 patients and 14 820 healthy controls in 52 countries (Fig. 1.3), Yusuf *et al.* (2004) found that being a current smoker compared with never being a smoker was the most important independent risk factor, increasing the risk of heart attack almost three times (2.87). Psychosocial stress, including depression, external locus of control, perceived stress and life events, was the second most important factor increasing the risk 2.67 times, followed by diabetes, hypertension and obesity. Regular moderate alcohol consumption, regular physical exercise and daily consumption of fruits and vegetables were associated with a significantly lowered risk (10–30%) of myocardial infarction.

As shown in the study by Yusuf *et al.* (2004), behavioural factors such as unhealthy food habits (fast food, fatty food, sugar, lack of vegetables and fruit), sedentary behaviour, and cigarette smoking, in addition to stress, contribute to cardiovascular risk. Regular physical activity, consumption of fruits and vegetables and moderate alcohol consumption are factors known to reduce the risk of cardiovascular disorders. High alcohol consumption and binge drinking, however, are associated with increased risk of CHD. Thus, these behavioural factors are important in themselves but are also known to be stress-related. Stress may have an indirect effect by contributing to the consumption of more fat and sugar as a result of reduced physical activity as a consequence of a lack of time to exercise or to prepare food that is more healthy; to increase cigarette smoking among smokers; and to increase alcohol consumption as a means of coping with high stress levels. If these indirect effects are included, this means that the importance of stress for the development of cardiovascular disorders (CVD) such as myocardial infarction and stroke may be even greater than indicated in the study by Yusuf *et al.* (2004) where the influence of psychosocial stress was controlled for other risk factors. An unhealthy lifestyle can hence be considered as both a cause of CVD and as caused by stressful conditions.

In a Canadian study, Aboa-Éboulé *et al.* (2007) investigated whether job strain increases the risk of recurrent CHD. In a prospective study, 972 men and women aged 35 to 59 years who returned to work after a first myocardial infarction were followed up between 1996 and 2005. Patients were interviewed 6 weeks after their return to work, then after 2 and 6 years. A measure of chronic job strain (high demands and low decision latitude) was constructed based on the first two interviews, and patients were divided into those exposed to high strain at both interviews and those unexposed to high strain at one or both interviews. It was found that patients exposed to chronic job strain after returning to work were twice as likely to have a second heart attack after 2.2 years of follow-up compared with those with less job strain.

CONCLUSION

A large body of scientific evidence shows that work-related stress is strongly linked to mental and physical health, including serious somatic diseases such as heart attacks (Theorell, 2008; Schnall *et al.*, 2009). Important questions are how the psychosocial work environment gets into the body, and what the mechanisms are that link mental stress to physical disorders. In order to understand these relationships, the influence of stress on bodily functions, behaviour and lifestyle needs to be analysed. In the next chapter we will describe how the brain interacts with the rest of the body in response to stress and how bodily responses to stress under certain circumstances promote health and protect the body but under other conditions can cause a wide variety of symptoms and health problems, including cardiovascular, metabolic, cognitive and musculoskeletal disorders (MSD). This information is necessary for prevention and interventions to promote health at work.

5 Responses to Stress

MIND–BODY INTERACTION

By tradition, and with roots in Cartesian philosophy, mind and body have been treated as separate entities. For example, until recently, mental disorders were treated by specialists in mental hospitals and bodily disorders in somatic hospitals. However, for a long time it has been known that mind and body interact continuously, with mental as well as physical consequences. That the brain is a very important part of the human body, and mental processes have a strong influence on various bodily functions and somatic symptoms, are obvious. People suffering from mental disorders, such as depression and anxiety, often present a number of physical symptoms such as diffuse pain, headache, gastrointestinal disorders, irregular heartbeat and dizziness. Similarly, physical symptoms and somatic disease may cause psychological disorders such as anxiety, depression, worry and sleeping problems. Such a mutual influence between mind and body could easily start a vicious circle with increasing mental and somatic symptoms. For example, pain syndromes will cause sleeping problems and lack of sleep, and insomnia in its turn will adversely affect the anabolic and regenerative processes in the body, impair immune functions and eventually increase pain sensitivity, which will have additional detrimental effects on sleep quality and amount of sleep.

Since the brain and other parts of the body are constantly communicating via a number of channels, interaction between what is happening in the brain and in the rest of the body seems natural (Fig. 5.1). Nerves send electrochemical signals from the brain to all parts of the body (efferent nerves), and the body sends signals via nerves to the brain (afferent nerves). Some of these signals are based on feedback loops in which signals from the brain affect bodily processes, for example blood pressure and heart rate, and the body sends signals back to inform the brain about conditions in the body. The brain sends signals that adjust blood pressure and heart rate to fit the actual and expected demands. For example, just standing up from bed requires a massive increase in blood pressure and heart rate and a redistribution of blood to ensure that the brain receives enough oxygen. Failure to do so would result in fainting or dizziness. An athlete preparing for a hundred-metre run has to mobilise all mental and physiological resources before the start in order to meet this challenge and be competitive.

The autonomic nervous system is of particular importance for regulating cardiovascular and neuroendocrine responses to stress. It consists of two main subparts, the sympathetic

The Science of Occupational Health: Stress, Psychobiology and the New World of Work, first edition
By Ulf Lundberg and Cary L. Cooper. Published 2011 by Blackwell Publishing Ltd
© 2011 Ulf Lundberg and Cary L. Cooper

Perceived stress influences the body

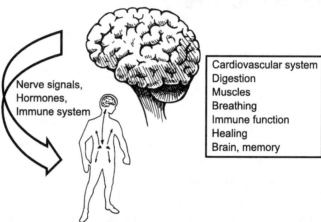

Fig. 5.1 The interaction of brain (mind) and body. Drawing by Urban Skytt.

nervous system (SNS) and the parasympathetic nervous system (PNS), which regulate various functions in opposition. Increased SNS activity stimulates heart rate, blood pressure and blood flow in the muscles whereas increased PNS has the opposite effect. Under normal conditions, activity of the SNS and PNS creates an optimal balance between activity, arousal and energy mobilisation ('fight or flight') on the one hand, and rest, recovery and energy storage on the other.

In addition to nerve signals, the brain communicates with the rest of the body via hormones secreted by glands in the brain into the blood stream. These hormones will execute their effects as soon as they find the correct receptor, which initiates functional changes in a physiological system or an organ (including other glands). The pituitary in the brain is one of the most important glands, and is under the influence of the hypothalamus which is the 'stress centre' of the brain. It secretes hormones regulating, among other things, stress responses, reproductive functions and growth. Glands in the body produce hormones which in some cases pass the blood–brain barrier and exert their effects on various brain functions. Examples are the stress hormone cortisol and the sex hormone oestrogen. Hormones complement nerve signals to help the brain to regulate various bodily systems according to environmental demands as well as internal needs. For example, physical conditions such as cold, heat and heavy physical demands will evoke activities in the body aimed at increasing coping resources and protecting the body. Cold induces shivering and physical activity, which help the body to increase its temperature, and heat induces widening of peripheral blood vessels and sweating, which reduce body temperature by losing heat via the skin. Physical demands increase heart rate and blood pressure, which allow more energy and oxygen to be transported to the muscles and the heart. The cortex of the brain receives signals from the environment via sensory organs (vision, sound, smell, etc.) and evaluates and interprets these signals and, on the basis of previous experiences, anticipates forthcoming demands and threats and prepares the body in advance for these events. This means that worrying about possible future threats and demands and ruminating about past events can keep the body aroused for long periods of time without actual or immediate threats.

Also the immune system serves as a communication system between the brain and the body. Its main job is to protect the body against viruses, bacteria, mycoses, foreign substances and abnormal and sick cells (e.g. cancer cells), and to contribute to the healing processes, but it also informs the brain about what is happening in the body. For example, when the body is infected by a virus, certain signal substances (cytokines) are secreted and execute their influence on the brain and the individual's condition. Cytokines make the individual feel unwell and tired, which is likely to serve an important function by preventing him or her from strenuous activities when ill thereby allowing the body to rest and use all its resources to fight the disease, contributing to a more rapid recovery. Cytokines also induce increased body temperature (fever), which contributes to killing bacteria and viruses in the body. Mental events, such as stress and physical activity, have an influence on the efficiency of the immune system and hence on susceptibility to infections, as illustrated in Chapter 6.

Mental processes, such as beliefs, attributions and conditioning, can induce intense somatic symptoms. For example, cancer patients undergoing chemotherapy often develop not only acute side effects but also anticipatory nausea and vomiting (Stockhurst *et al.*, 2006), which is likely to be acquired by Pavlovian conditioning. Nausea and vomiting are symptoms that very rapidly become conditioned to a stimulus, and consequently anything associated with the treatment may be conditioned to nausea. The patient may react with nausea or vomiting by just seeing the nurse providing the chemotherapy, or the clinic or even the hospital building (Hursti, 1994). Another example is those people who are convinced that exposure to electromagnetic fields from mobile phones and other electrical equipment induces symptoms such as skin complaints (redness, burning sensations), fatigue, headache, dizziness, nausea and increased pulse. However, in a number of controlled experiments it has been shown that individuals with these problems cannot distinguish between real exposure to such fields and sham exposure, and that symptoms appear only when they 'think' that they are exposed, regardless of actual exposure. Hillert *et al.* (2008) exposed 38 symptomatic and 33 non-symptomatic individuals to 3 hours of radio-frequency fields and sham exposure, in a randomised order with a 1-week interval in a double-blind study. A belief that radio-frequency fields were active was associated with skin symptoms in the symptomatic group, but neither group could detect the fields better than chance. When individuals are exposed to environmental conditions that coincide with or precede certain symptoms, a natural human reaction is to interpret that as a causal relation. This makes the symptoms more understandable and creates a sense of comprehensibility (Antonovsky, 1987). If this association is correct, it also helps the individual to avoid exposure to similar adverse conditions in the future. If it is not correct, this attribution may induce symptoms just by being exposed to the assumed agent.

The three important communication systems between the brain (mind) and the body, i.e. nerves, hormones and the immune system, work both independently and together and influence all important bodily functions and systems. The most important systems and processes in the body influenced by mental processes are the neuroendocrine (nerves and hormones), cardiovascular (heart, blood vessels, blood), gastrointestinal (saliva, stomach, intestines, metabolism) and immune systems, the muscles and sleep. Functional disturbances in these systems, reflected in symptoms and diseases such as cardiovascular and metabolic disorders, infections, pain symptoms and sleeping problems, can be caused by perceived stress and other mental processes.

THE NEUROENDOCRINE STRESS SYSTEMS

Two neuroendocrine systems are of particular importance in response to stress, the sympathetic adrenal medullary (SAM) system, with the secretion of the two catecholamines,

Environmental demands trigger the release of hormones

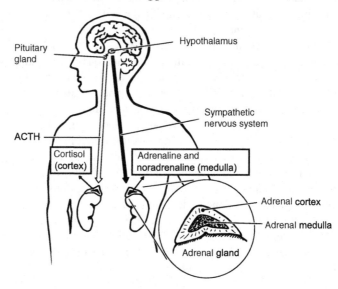

Fig. 5.2   The two major stress systems. Drawing by Urban Skytt.

adrenaline and noradrenaline; and the hypothalamic pituitary adrenocortical (HPA) system with the secretion of corticosteroids (Fig. 5.2). Cortisol is the most important corticosteroid in the human stress response. Corticosterone serves a similar role in certain other animals, e.g. rats.

The hypothalamus is the stress centre of the brain, regulating activity in the pituitary gland and the autonomic nervous system, and thus the stress responses. When an individual perceives or anticipates an acute stress situation, the cortex of the brain sends signals to the hypothalamus, which will activate a cascade of events in the body relevant for coping with stress. First, the SNS is activated and sends nerve signals to the adrenal medulla, which responds by secreting the stress hormones adrenaline and noradrenaline, also known as catecholamines, into the blood stream. This is a rapid response (less than a minute), and is of particular importance for coping with acute short-term stress. Secretion of adrenaline and noradrenaline into the blood stream increases heart rate and blood pressure, which means that more blood with nutrients and oxygen can be transported to the muscles, the heart and the brain and prepare the individual for 'battle'. The catecholamines also stimulate the release of glucose and free fatty acids from the liver (lipolysis) and hence increase the amount of energy in the blood. During acute stress, digesting food (metabolic activity) would take too long to produce the energy needed immediately. Metabolic activity contributes to long-term energy storage, but would in an acute situation tax bodily resources and reduce the individual's capacity to combat the stressor. As a consequence, evolution has caused these processes to slow down during acute stress.

Noradrenaline is released from the adrenal medulla but is also a transmitter substance in the SNS, sending signals from one neuron to another via synapses. When these neurons are active, noradrenaline leaks out from the synapse sites and therefore the major part of noradrenaline in the blood comes from sympathetic nerve endings. Physical activity and changes in body posture involve activity of the SNS, and are thus reflected in increased release of noradrenaline into the blood. As a consequence, secretion of noradrenaline is more closely linked to 'physical' stress, whereas adrenaline secretion from the adrenal medulla is mainly influenced by 'mental' stress. A certain fraction of the circulating catecholamines is excreted into the urine, which makes it possible to measure the levels of these stress hormones not only in blood but also from urine samples.

The other main physiological stress system, the HPA axis, is also controlled by the hypothalamus and other parts of the brain, such as the hippocampal formation. In response to stress, hormonal signals are sent from the hypothalamus and hippocampus to the anterior pituitary, which secretes another hormone, adrenocorticotropic hormone (ACTH), which via the blood stream reaches the adrenal cortex where it exerts its effects. The adrenal cortex responds by increased release of cortisol into the blood. This process is much slower than the neural (SNS) regulation of the adrenal medulla. It takes about half an hour for cortisol secretion to reach its peak level in response to a stressful situation. Thus, cortisol is of particular importance for adaptation to long-term or chronic stress by influencing the metabolism in all cells in the body, the storage of fat, the activity of the immune system and certain brain functions (e.g. memory).

Animal studies by Meaney (2001) and colleagues (Francis *et al.*, 1999) have demonstrated how early environmental regulation of gene expression and brain development influences behavioural and endocrine responses to stress. The kind of care a mother gives to her offspring also determines the animal's responses to stress in adulthood. For example, animals who receive less grooming and licking when born produce more stress hormones when exposed to challenging stress situations, which later in life may increase the risk of heart disease and diabetes. From an evolutionary perspective, this early programming of stress systems is likely to be of importance for survival in a physically harsh world but is inadequate if the demands mainly consist of mental challenges. These mechanisms have been demonstrated experimentally in animal studies. In view of the similarities between the physiological stress systems in humans and animals, there are reasons to believe that similar factors also operate in humans. Humans, however, need much more time than rats to develop into adults, and are thus more open to environmental influences during infancy, childhood and adolescence and have bigger brains and more advanced cognitive skills. Humans are therefore likely to be more adaptive to later environmental influences than rats, but research consistently shows that conditions in early life (pre- and postnatal) are of great importance for human adult well-being, health and life expectancy.

In chronic long-term stress, compared with acute short-term stress, the bodily consequences of activation of the stress systems differ as described in more detail below. In general, chronic stress causes health problems because the stress responses, which are protective from a short-term perspective, become a threat to the body when they are sustained over long periods of time.

THE CARDIOVASCULAR SYSTEM

The cardiovascular system, that is, the heart, the blood and the blood vessels in all parts of the body, is regulated by the autonomic nervous system, which distributes oxygen and nutrients to the cells and removes waste products away from the cells. The heart is the pump running this system, which first sends blood to the lungs to pick up oxygen from breathing air and then pumps the oxygenated (arterial) blood to the rest of the body, including the heart itself.

Increased sympathetic activity raises heart rate and contributes to vasoconstriction of the blood vessels transporting blood to the muscles and the brain. This increases blood pressure and the speed of transportation of blood to the effector organs, whereas elevated parasympathetic activity will reduce heart rate and blood pressure. In conclusion, raised heart rate may be caused by elevated sympathetic as well as reduced parasympathetic activity. During stress, sympathetic activity will dominate over parasympathetic activity, and is reflected in increased heart rate and reduced heart rate variability.

A proper regulation of the cardiovascular system is necessary for adequate adaptation and coping with various mental and physical demands. In response to physical demands, activation of the cardiovascular system is necessary for survival. However, during mental stress when physical activity is low, chronic overactivity of the cardiovascular system will increase the risk of cardiovascular disorders such as atherosclerosis, hypertension, heart attack (myocardial infarction) and stroke.

High blood pressure (hypertension) is an important risk factor for heart attack. Menkes *et al.* (1989) investigated the relation between blood pressure reactivity to stress in about 1000 medical students and development of high blood pressure for up to 40 years later. When entering medical school at the age of about 20, students were exposed to a test of stress reactivity, the cold pressor test (placing a hand in ice-cold water), and the increase in blood pressure compared with that at rest was measured. The students were followed up for a period of 20 to 40 years by recording the development of hypertension (medical diagnosis or medication against high blood pressure). By a median split on the basis of systolic blood pressure responses to stress at the age of 20, high- and low-reactivity groups were formed. No differences in hypertension were found during the first 20 years, but after this period the high-reactivity group started to develop high blood pressure to a much greater extent than did the low-reactivity group. This means that elevated stress reactivity at the age of 20 can predict increased risk of hypertension 20 years later.

COPING WITH STRESS

In order to understand the role of stress responses today, it is important to keep in mind that bodily responses to stress in humans and animals have developed during evolution over millions of years, and contributed to survival and protection of the body in a world that was changing very slowly. The stress responses are mainly adequate as a means for preparing the body for battle by giving the individual extra strength, physically and mentally, when this is needed. Different species, such as fish, birds and mammals, including humans, respond similarly to stress. In animals, evolutionary principles are still of importance and contribute to survival of the fittest, but have less influence over human adaptation and survival.

Natural selection depends largely on the existence of considerable individual variation in characteristics within species. Under slowly changing environmental conditions, certain individuals who are better fitted to the new situation will have a greater chance of survival and of spreading their genes to their offspring and coming generations, which successively can adapt to slowly changing conditions by natural selection. Under more rapidly changing conditions, such as those that humans have experienced during the last two millennia, evolutionary adaptation is not possible. Evolution also depends on mutations, which are sudden changes in genes (DNA). However, mutations are often harmful rather than beneficial for survival, and therefore do not constitute a reliable means to ensure survival of endangered species in a rapidly changing world.

One example of how rapid environmental changes can cause disasters for certain species is the extinction of the dinosaurs about 65 million years ago. After having dominated the Earth for more than 160 million years, the dinosaurs and about 70% of all the species on the Earth at that time died during a relatively short period of time (from an evolutionary perspective). One likely explanation is that the Earth was hit by a giant asteroid/meteorite, which changed the climate dramatically. No subgroup of dinosaurs had the characteristics necessary to survive and reproduce for a longer period of time under these new conditions, and time was too short for beneficial mutations to occur. Rapid climate changes are also taking place today. The greenhouse effect and the changing climate on the Earth leading to the melting of ice sheets in the North (Greenland) and the South (Antarctic) are one important example. This ongoing change is likely to put pressure on a number of species and increase their risk of extinction unless they are protected by adequate intervention. For example, polar bears are endangered and at risk of extinction due to a shrinking Arctic ice shelf which reduces their chances of finding food (hunting seals) and places for mating. This development forces them to swim longer and longer distances from the shore to reach the ice, with risk of drowning.

In conclusion, human beings today are roughly the same biological individuals as their ancestors were a hundred thousand years ago. This means that we respond to threats and stress by activating the same systems in the body as did Stone Age man (Fig. 5.3). In many cases this is still an adequate response, but under many circumstances these responses are inadequate and may cause disturbances of body functions, especially when they are prolonged. Conflicting demands, unclear instructions, an irritating boss, economic problems, an insecure occupational position and risk of unemployment, dissatisfaction with colleagues and work tasks, too complex or too many problems to solve, tight deadlines, etc., are problems that cannot be solved by elevated physical strength, high blood pressure and heart rate, release of blood lipids and glucose. When this mobilisation of energy cannot be used for fight or flight, it may damage the cardiovascular system and increase the atherosclerotic process and blood clotting. Most individuals are relatively robust and can resist short periods of high stress levels without health problems, but long-term stress, even at a moderate level, is harmful. As mental stress in terms of worrying, ruminating about past events and anticipation of future threats cannot be shut off in the same way as physical activity can be, it is likely to be of particular importance for chronic stress exposure and concomitant health problems.

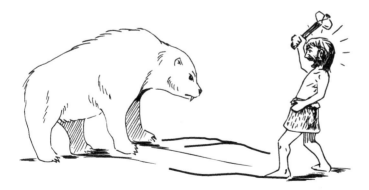

Fig. 5.3   The human body is prepared for battle (fight-or-flight response). Drawing by Urban Skytt.

Why zebras don't get ulcers

In his book, *Why Zebras Don't Get Ulcers*, Sapolsky (1998) summarises findings on the role of stress in a number of disorders. His main aim is to emphasise the important role of 'rest and recovery' for long-term health. Zebras are used as symbols for how animals differ from humans in their way of coping with stress. On the savannah, zebras are repeatedly exposed to severe stress in terms of being chased by lions and other predatory animals. They have to run for their lives. In this situation, the lion's and the zebra's stress systems are activated to a maximum in order to run as fast as possible to survive (to eat or not to be eaten). Life or death depends on how successful the animals are in terms of mobilising their extra resources. The chase does not last very long. If the zebra is faster, the lion soon gives up its attack and the zebra also stops running and returns rapidly to more productive activities, such as eating, mating and sleeping. In contrast, human beings exposed to a similar threat to their lives would not be able to relax after the attack, enjoy a good meal, sleep or have intercourse. Humans would probably be in shock and would feel intense distress about the event for days, weeks or months and ruminate about what could have happened ('I could have been killed and eaten by a lion'), and also worry about the risk of similar attacks on their life in the future. This means that their stress systems would be kept activated for long periods of time, consequently increasing the risk of causing dysregulation of important bodily systems and the development of stress-related disorders. According to Sapolsky, zebras and other animals are better able than humans to shut off their extraordinary responses to an acute stress situation as soon as the threat is over, and consequently do not develop stress-related health problems to the same extent as do humans. However, he also points out that animals living under unnatural conditions, such as in small cages at a zoo or being transported long distances under crowded conditions, often develop stress-related symptoms. This emphasises the importance of compensating stressful periods with time for rest, recovery and restitution in order to stay healthy.

Sapolsky has chosen stomach ulcers as an example of a stress-related disorder. Today, some people may question the role of stress in the development of ulcers because a bacterium, *Helicobacter pylori*, has been found to be involved. However, more than 50% of people harbour this bacterium but are asymptomatic, which indicates that other factors are involved too. The possible role of stress for this disease is discussed in Chapter 6.

ACUTE STRESS

Stress hormones

The sensory organs (vision, hearing, touch) inform the brain (cortex) about threatening conditions in the environment and in response the cortex signals to the hypothalamus and hippocampus in the brain to prepare the body for battle. Just thinking about a stressful situation may elicit a similar response. The physiological stress systems described above are activated via neural and hormonal signals, and increased amounts of adrenaline, noradrenaline and cortisol are secreted into the blood. Bodily resources are mobilised through elevated heart rate and blood pressure, a redistribution of blood from the gastrointestinal system and the skin in favour of the muscles and the brain, and a release of energy in terms of lipids and glucose from the liver. These responses are accompanied by mental experiences such as focused attention and feelings of stress, tenseness, anxiety, fear and aggression. The intensity of the subjective experiences of stress is related to the magnitude of the physiological stress responses. For example, during normal work conditions, adrenaline and noradrenaline levels increase 50–100% compared with non-work conditions (Lundberg & Johansson, 2000), whereas intensely stressful situations, such as childbirth and defence of a doctoral dissertation, may induce stress hormone levels that are more than ten times higher than normal. Adrenaline secretion is mainly related to mental stress intensity, whereas noradrenaline is more strongly related to physical demands and body posture. This means that manual workers usually have a higher level of noradrenaline compared with white-collar workers.

The normal circadian variation in cortisol includes a peak in the morning about 30 minutes after waking up. The magnitude of this increase seems to depend on previous experiences, including sleep, as well as on anticipated demands. Lack of recovery and bad sleep during the night are associated with elevated cortisol levels in the morning, which can be seen as compensatory mechanisms helping the individual to cope with daily activities despite lack of restitution. In the short term this is beneficial, but sustained lack of rest will be harmful.

During very intense stress, both catecholamine and cortisol levels increase considerably, with the two major stress systems supporting each other in order to help the individual to cope. One example is childbirth. During the period of labour, catecholamine and cortisol levels in women increase 400–600% compared with their normal pregnancy levels at the same time of the day (Alehagen et al., 2001). During the last phase of pushing, with the full opening of the uterus and the infant ready to leave the mother's body, cortisol levels in a group of mothers were found to be on average about 11 times higher than during pregnancy (Alehagen et al., 2005). For individual mothers, much higher levels were recorded. Perceived pain and fear on a group level followed the increase in cortisol and adrenaline levels. For women receiving pain relief in terms of epidural analgesia, pain, fear and cortisol levels were much lower but adrenaline and cortisol levels were still 400–500% higher than during pregnancy.

Compared with stress levels at work, the stress hormone output of women during childbirth is extreme, but probably necessary for coping successfully with the intense mental and physical demands facing women during labour. However, a difference between childbirth and normal work is that childbirth happens a few times in a woman's life and lasts for a relatively short period of time, usually less than 24 hours. No one would be able to endure stress hormone levels ten times the normal level for a longer period of time without serious health consequences. Going to work is something that happens to most people five days a week, week after week and year after year, and there is strong evidence that even moderate levels of stress lasting for long periods of time will cause health problems sooner or later. An example of how extreme stress may destroy the body can be found in salmon fighting against streams and waterfalls to reach their place of birth upstream to spawn. Soon after spawning they die as a result of the extremely high levels of stress hormones (corticosteroids such as cortisol) which have caused lesions, infections and a complete breakdown of their immune system.

Pain

Pain sensitivity is regulated by peripheral as well as central (CNS) mechanisms (Wolf & Salter, 2000), including psychological factors (Price, 2000). In response to stress, pain signals are attenuated or blocked, which means that the individual can focus on reducing stress by eliminating the threat without being influenced by pain from possible injuries. This is a great advantage in stress situations, where fight or flight is necessary for survival. The individual can continue to fight or run away from the scene without being hampered by pain.

Examples are soldiers who are badly injured during combat but do not notice their condition until the fight is over. Intensive competition in sport induces similar effects. In boxing, for instance, injuries are common yet do not interfere with participants' performance. It is usually up to the referee to judge when it is time to stop the fight because one of the fighters is badly injured. In other forms of sport, such as football, one would expect a similar phenomenon in a player who has just been tackled, but for some reason the player may sometimes behave as if the pain is unbearable — especially if the incident occurs close to the goal. However, the player usually recovers rapidly if a penalty kick is given. Reduced pain sensitivity during stress is to some extent beneficial in modern society but could also, for example, contribute to more extensive exposure to health hazards under stressful work conditions. The immediate negative effects of heat, cold, noise, pollution, non-ergonomic work positions and heavy lifting may not be noticed at times of intense stress but may cause damage and pain later on.

Blood coagulation

Blood coagulation increases during stress and the blood becomes 'stickier'. This reduces bleeding in the event of wounding and increases the chances of survival in a fight. In response to psychosocial stress, increased coagulation can be harmful and increases the risk of thrombosis. Thrombosis is the formation of a blood clot that obstructs the flow of blood through the circulatory system and may migrate from one part of the body (embolism) and cause a blockage of a blood vessel in another part. Blood clotting in the blood vessels supporting the heart (coronary arteries) would cause a myocardial infarction. In a review of the literature on blood coagulation and fibrinolysis, von Känel *et al.* (2001) concluded that psychological factors such as mental stress activate coagulation and fibrinolysis and that this constitutes a possible pathway to coronary artery disease. Von Känel *et al.* (2009) also investigated job stress and coagulation measures in blood (plasma) in 52 healthy teachers and found that overcommitment predicted increased coagulability after recovery from stress.

Immune responses

In response to short-term stress, such as mental, physical or infectious challenges, the activity of the immune system is enhanced. This protects the body from invasion of foreign cells, viruses and bacteria and speeds up the process of wound healing. However, this is a short-term enhancement of the immune system. When stress continues, this response is followed by a successive decline in immune responsiveness and a concomitant increased susceptibility to infections. As demonstrated by Dhabhar and McEwen (1997), acute stress enhances immune functions whereas chronic stress suppresses them.

Overactivation of the immune system, for example as a result of repeated acute stress exposure, may also cause health problems in terms of increasing the risk of autoimmune diseases such as multiple sclerosis, juvenile (Type 1) diabetes, rheumatoid arthritis, asthma and allergies. In these cases, the inflammatory responses are chronic and the immune system also attacks and destroys healthy cells such as the insulin-producing cells in the pancreas, which is the cause of Type 1 diabetes. A period of overactivity in a physiological system is often followed by a 'rebound effect', that is, a period of underactivity. With regard to the immune system, this could explain a phenomenon reported by many that infections such as the common cold often appear just after, rather than during, a period of stress.

Digestion and mobilisation of energy

Metabolic activity to digest food is not prioritised in an acute stress situation. This is a slow process to provide the energy that is needed immediately. The energy required to cope with an acute stress situation will be released more rapidly from sources within the body, such as the liver, in terms of free fatty acids and glucose to the working muscles, the brain and the heart. Digestion to produce and store energy would tax the individual's resources in an acute situation and is therefore postponed until the stress is over. Therefore, all parts of the metabolic system are deactivated during stress, such as saliva production (leading to a dry mouth) and activity in the stomach and the intestines. As a consequence, a nervous speaker usually needs a glass of water to compensate for the reduced saliva production. Employees under stress at work are usually not particularly hungry, and may take just a short lunch break with fast food or will eat while working.

The rate of CHD is about 50% higher among men in Sweden compared with men in France. In the Renault–Volvo heart project (Simon *et al.*, 1997; Kumlin *et al.*, 2001), samples of about 1000 automotive workers from Renault, France, and Volvo, Sweden, were compared in terms of lifestyle factors. In general the French workers had a greater number of traditional risk factors for CHD (smoking, overweight, higher-fat diet). However, French workers reported eating more vegetables, drinking more red wine and spending significantly more time on having lunch and dinner compared with the Swedish workers. The causal relationship between these differences in lifestyle and CHD is not clear, but it is possible that spending more time on meals reduces stress and promotes digestion, which, combined with the higher consumption of red wine and vegetables, counteracts some of the negative effects of smoking on CHD risk (Yusuf *et al.*, 2004).

Cognitive functions: 'tunnel vision'

Stress also has important cognitive effects, inducing 'tunnel vision'. This means that all attention is focused on the immediate threat and peripheral signals are ignored. This is likely to have been of importance for survival under physical threats by helping the individual to focus on the most immediate challenge. Today, however, tunnel vision may under certain conditions be a risk factor by contributing to accidents or economic costs as a result of ignoring important peripheral information. In traffic, for instance, tunnel vision may cause the missing of peripheral signals such as a red light, a car coming from behind or a pedestrian crossing the street, which may result in fatal accidents. In occupational and political decision making under time pressure, tunnel vision may cause the neglect of important background information with costly consequences. Examples are the ignorance of contra-indications for surgery in medical decisions, mistakes due to not double checking the dose of medication, firefighters not investigating the possible presence of explosives in a building they are to enter, and decisions about an organisation's or a company's future strategy without including relevant information about ongoing changes in the market and customer preferences. Tunnel vision or the narrowing of the attention span occurring under stress may hence cause decisions to be made on the basis of information that is limited or biased.

Cognitive functions: memory and conditioning

Certain memory functions are strengthened under acute stress. This is of importance for helping individuals to remember how they got involved in a life-threatening situation. By remembering how mistakes were made that led to a critical situation or a serious accident, the individual would have a better chance of avoiding similar situations in the future. As a consequence of this phenomenon, most people remember the circumstances associated with events that induced strong emotions and stressful experiences. For example, most people remember what they were doing, where they were and how they received information about the attack on the World Trade Centre in New York in 2001. A sudden and unexpected death of a close family member or information about diagnosis of serious disease induces a similar effect on memory. People usually remember how they learned that their mother or father had a heart attack, or under what conditions they were told by their doctor that they had cancer. These effects are immediate and 'automatic', and do not need time to be spent on practising to remember. These memories also seem to be very long-lasting. People who experienced the murder of President John F. Kennedy in Dallas in 1963 usually still remember how they learned about this event, where they were at that moment and what they were doing. (One of the authors of this book is among them and still remembers how he learned about the event from newspaper headlines on his way one morning to a psychology examination at the university.) Thus, acute stress contributes to processes in the brain that improve the storage of information about important events. At work the experience of strong emotional reactions could be health protective, for example by enabling the more efficient storage of information about the conditions that caused or nearly caused a serious accident. However, if strong negative reactions have been linked to a manager, co-workers or other conditions at the workplace, not being able to forget these circumstances may induce a generalised negative attitude towards the job. Low job satisfaction is known to increase the risk of CHD and MSD.

Animals respond in a similar way and remember when they have experienced dangerous and unpleasant situations, which increases their chances of survival. For example, a rat that becomes ill from eating food with rat poison will never eat the same food again. Rats are usually very cautious and first taste only a small piece of unfamiliar food to find out what happens. To overcome this strategy, rat poison has been developed which affects and kills the animal long after eating, which reduces the rat's chances of making an association between eating a particular kind of food and becoming ill. Most parents find that small children are very suspicious about eating new kinds of food. This is likely to have been of importance for health and survival from an evolutionary perspective, by protecting them from poisonous and unhealthy food. Nausea is a very strong conditioning stimulus for humans and animals. Feeling sick in one's stomach creates a very strong association with items present at the same time. For example, vomiting after having eaten a particular kind of food would cause an aversion to it for a long period of time, and mere exposure to the smell of it might evoke nausea even if the food was not the reason for vomiting.

An acute alarm system

Physiological stress reactions are usually regulated by perceived stress (i.e. conscious cognitive thoughts in the brain): "Will I be able to cope with this situation or not?" However, the body also seems to have an acute alarm system, a very quick mechanism that triggers stress responses even before the individual is consciously aware of the threat. A sudden unfamiliar sound in a quiet room, or noticing a movement nearby in a situation in which you think that you are alone, would first cause a few seconds of reduced heart rate during the initial intake of the information ('My heart stopped beating from fear'), followed by a rapid increase in heart rate and mobilisation of resources for fight or flight. If the cognitive process that follows the immediate reaction concludes that it was a 'false alarm', the stress response will vanish and biological functions will return to normal. Öhman and Soares (1994) tested the hypothesis that unconscious exposure to phobic stimuli is sufficient to elicit human fear responses. They found that snake- and spider-fearful participants exposed to phobic (snakes, spiders) and control pictures (flowers, mushrooms) showed elevated sympathetic responses (increased skin conductance) to snake and spider pictures as compared with neutral pictures without being consciously aware of the exposure. This rapid alarm system without conscious cognitive processing is probably very important for animals hunted by predators, who can start running or flying away rapidly when they hear a sudden noise or see a moving shadow, without having to evaluate the signals and decide whether they are exposed to a real threat or not. In humans, unconscious rapid reactions can under certain conditions cause serious mistakes and accidents.

Stage fright and vicious mind–body interactions

Bodily responses to stress such as increased heart rate can also contribute to intensified feelings of stress and initiate a vicious circle. For example, a speaker or an artist who is performing in front of an audience and feels his or her heart pounding may become even more stressed, which could impair performance. Feeling more stressed would induce an even higher heart rate, followed by more intense feelings of stress, worse performance and so on. Intense stress impairs performance by narrowing the attention and inducing disorganised behaviour. Methods to break this vicious circle can involve relaxation training, with applied techniques of breathing in order to relax rapidly and physical activity, but other common methods for coping with stress-induced high heart rate include intake of alcohol and medication with betablockers.

Summary of bodily responses to acute stress

- Increased secretion of stress hormones.
- Increased blood pressure and heart rate.
- Decreased digestion and reproductive activity.
- Release of glucose and free fatty acids from the liver.
- Increased immune activity.
- Decreased pain sensitivity.
- Increased coagulation.
- Tunnel vision.
- Enhanced memory.
- Increased performance (fight or flight).

In summary, an individual exposed to acute stress may show a high heart rate, high blood pressure, a dry mouth, pale or white skin and a narrow span of attention. The responses to acute stress induce a mobilisation of energy, which is helpful for survival in situations where force, speed and focused attention are of particular importance. However, in response to psychosocial and mental stress where physical strength is not an adequate means of coping, increased blood pressure, heart rate, and coagulation and elevated levels of blood lipids are harmful rather than protective by increasing the risk of CVD as described in Chapter 6. In general, however, short-term or acute stress is associated with several beneficial effects, such as improved performance, memory and immune function, and reduced pain sensitivity, and does not constitute a major health problem.

CHRONIC STRESS

In contrast to the acute stress responses, long-term or chronic stress often induces the opposite effects. Chronic stress is usually associated with impaired performance, memory and immune functions, and increased pain sensitivity. Negative emotions during prolonged stress, such as anxiety, distress, dissatisfaction, sadness and depression, tax the individual's executive functions and reduce his or her capacity to work efficiently. High job satisfaction and psychological well-being, on the other hand, are associated with good performance. Not only chronic mental stress but also excessive long-term physical demands can cause impaired performance. Kentää (2001) investigated overtraining, staleness and burnout in sports, and concluded that too much training, high levels of psychosocial stress and lack of recovery accounted for the majority of these disorders in athletes. Overtraining has many similarities to mentally induced stress conditions such as burnout and chronic fatigue syndromes.

In chronic stress, the role of the stress hormone cortisol becomes particularly important. For normal healthy functioning, cortisol levels should be regulated according to internal and external needs. This is done via feedback loops in the hypothalamus and hippocampus. Production of too little cortisol is therefore also a health problem. Cortisol has anti-inflammatory effects, and balances the effects of the immune system. An overactive immune system causes autoimmune diseases such as allergies, asthma and rheumatoid arthritis. The immune system overreacts to harmless things such as dust, pollen and pet dander, and joints can be chronically inflamed. Other serious autoimmune diseases include systemic lupus erythematosus (SLE), in which the immune system attacks the body's cells and tissue, resulting in inflammation and tissue damage, and multiple sclerosis, a degenerative disease in which the immune system destroys part of the nervous system. Pain is part of the inflammatory response of the immune system, and chronically low cortisol levels mean that inflammatory disorders are not kept under control. Inflammation can be suppressed by cortisone, a steroid hormone related to cortisol and corticosterone.

Cortisol effects the metabolism in the cells and contributes to an accumulation of fat in the abdominal region for two main reasons. First, there is a high density of cortisol receptors on the fat cells in the abdomen. When there is a surplus of energy in the body from carbohydrates, protein and fat in the food, this energy is stored as fat mainly in the central parts of the body when the individual is exposed to chronic stress and high cortisol levels. This is a protective factor securing access to energy under long-term stress, but chronic stress also reduces the production of anabolic hormones such as sex (oestrogen, testosterone) and growth hormones, which are important for regeneration and growth. Reduced levels of oestrogen in women, as happens rapidly after menopause, cause a redistribution of fat in the body. Fat stored on hips and thighs before menopause tends to move to the abdominal region. Similarly, reduced levels of testosterone in men, for example with increasing age, are associated with reduced muscle mass and accumulation of abdominal fat. The dominance of catabolic stress hormones such as cortisol, and reduced production of anabolic hormones under chronic stress, thus make male and female bodies more similar with age, with slimmer hips and legs and increased abdomen. In conclusion, chronic stress contributes to biological ageing. Ishizaki et al. (2008) investigated the effect of changes in psychosocial workplace characteristics on weight gain and abdominal obesity in 2200 men and 1371 women aged 30–53 years working in a factory. They found that high job strain according to the Demand–Control model is a risk factor for increased abdominal obesity. Reduction of stress exposure, regular physical exercise and weight loss, on the other hand, are known to reduce insulin resistance and the metabolic risk factors.

Chronic exposure to stress reduces the efficiency of the immune system, which means increased susceptibility to infections. As the immune system is also of importance in healing processes, wounds heal more slowly under stress. A number of controlled experiments have been performed to illustrate these effects and some of them are described in Chapter 6.

In an acute stress situation, pain signals are attenuated or blocked whereas long-term stress causes lower pain threshold and an increase in pain sensitivity. One example is the fibromyalgia syndrome (FMS), considered to be associated with chronic stress exposure. FMS patients show not only increased pain sensitivity at a number of tender points, but also generalised pain sensitivity (Petzke *et al.*, 2003). As chronic pain is a form of stress, this means that pain patients may become more and more pain sensitive. This is likely to create a vicious circle with increasing pain problems and eventually chronic illness. This increase in pain sensitivity is probably due to both peripheral factors (more sensitive pain receptors and more efficient communication of pain signals to the brain) and central factors (increased pain sensitivity in the brain). Pain receptors that have been irritated become more sensitive to new stimulation. Many individuals, for instance, find that exposure to too much sun makes the skin red and very sensitive. Just a light touch or normal clothing can in this situation be enough to induce intense pain. Cognitive factors, such as catastrophic thoughts ('I will never get better, my life is ruined by my pain'), are also of importance. By focusing on the pain, feeling helpless and anticipating a life-long pain condition, the pain gets worse and eventually creates a chronic handicap (Linton, 2002). Vervoort *et al.* (2006) measured pain catastrophising and negative affectivity in schoolchildren and children with chronic pain as related to pain, disability and somatic complaints. It was found that pain catastrophising significantly accounted for the variance of pain, disability and somatic complaints beyond the effects of age, sex and negative affectivity. Expectation that pain is harmless or will soon be over reduces the pain sensation. Treatment with placebo instead of a real painkiller may significantly reduce pain, and toothache is often diminished or eliminated just by entering the dentist's waiting room and knowing that help is near. Similarly, stressful work conditions are more easy to cope with when a holiday is approaching.

Episodic or personal memory functions are to a large extent located in the hippocampal formation in the brain. In response to chronic stress, the individual is exposed to high cortisol levels for a long period of time. This starts the degeneration of connections (dendrites) between neurons in the hippocampus, which also reduces the size of this region (Sapolsky, 1996; McEwen & Lasley, 2002). More information on this effect will be presented in Chapter 6. In a recent experimental animal study (Dias-Ferreira *et al.*, 2009), it was demonstrated that chronic stress also leads to bias in behavioural strategies. Rats exposed to chronic stress were found to shift towards habitual rather than goal-directed strategies. This means that chronic stress makes it difficult to inhibit a habit and respond appropriately in a decision-making situation. If these results are transferred to humans, this means that chronic stress could have serious negative consequences for people in decision-making positions by making them more likely to respond according to previous habits rather than making decisions which are adequate in a new situation.

Summary of bodily responses to chronic stress

- Dysregulation of stress responses.
- Hypertension (chronically elevated blood pressure).
- Atherosclerosis (clogged arteries).
- Metabolic disturbance, accumulation of abdominal fat.

- Impaired immune function.
- Increased pain sensitivity.
- Impaired memory function.
- Decreased performance.

SHORT-TERM VERSUS LONG-TERM STRESS

Elevated arousal or stress levels mean activation of bodily and mental resources, which helps the individual to cope with daily demands. In the short term, increased stress hormone levels of 50–100% are not a health problem. Stress hormone levels can increase much more when necessary, as illustrated by the high levels found during childbirth (Alehagen *et al.*, 2001), and among parachute trainees (Ursin *et al.*, 1978). This dramatic mobilisation of energy is also necessary for survival, and for coping with very demanding situations. However, when these extraordinary resources are no longer needed, it is equally important to shut off the stress responses, to unwind and let biological activity return to baseline levels, and allow time for rest and recovery and for anabolic processes aimed at regenerating resources. This is in line with the Allostatic Load model described below. Very intense stress levels, as displayed by women during labour, are important for coping with acute demands, but would be a serious threat to health if the response were prolonged as illustrated by salmon striving against the stream to spawn and the *karoshi* phenomenon in Japan. The regulation of important bodily functions is seriously disturbed if intense stress activation lasts for a longer period of time, as seen in people with post-traumatic stress disorder (PTSD), chronic fatigue, burnout and fibromyalgia syndrome (FMS). Depending on individual differences in vulnerability, general health status and coping resources, the intensity and duration of stress that may cause harm vary considerably between individuals. However, even moderate levels of stress would in the long term cause health problems in most people.

There is no clear distinction between short-term and long-term stress. Changes in regulatory functions occur gradually when individuals are exposed to repeated or chronic stress. A moderate response to mild stress is replaced by a more pronounced response during intense stress. Long-term exposure to intense stress seems to cause a dysregulation of the HPA axis and an attenuated cortisol response. Very intense stress, for example that associated with traumatic life events such as war, violence, rape and torture, may cause dysregulation of the HPA axis and mental and somatic health problems within days or weeks, whereas moderate work-related stress may continue for years until stress-related health problems start to appear. Llabre & Hadi (2009) performed a longitudinal study of Kuwaiti children exposed to war-related trauma during the Iraqi occupation and the Gulf War in 1993. On follow-up in 2003 they found a direct relationship between exposure and poor sleep quality and body mass index. Exposure to war-related events during childhood was also associated with post-traumatic stress and poor self-reported health in adulthood.

IMPORTANCE OF SLEEP

The long-term balance between stress/activity and rest/recovery is of significant importance for health outcomes. Sleep is the most important form of rest and recovery. Lack of sleep seems to induce a compensatory increase in cortisol secretion in the morning, which helps the individual to cope. In the short term this is not a problem, but long-term sleep deprivation will cause metabolic disturbances and health problems. For example, Cohen and colleagues (2009) recently demonstrated that individuals sleeping less than 7 hours a night who were exposed to nasal drops containing a rhinovirus had a threefold higher risk of developing upper respiratory infections (the common cold) compared with individuals sleeping 8 hours.

The quality of sleep seems even more important. Individuals sleeping less than 92% of the time in bed have more than five times as high a risk of becoming ill compared with individuals sleeping more than 98% of the time in bed. Slow-wave (deep) sleep is considered the most restorative form of sleep. Tasali *et al.* (2008) investigated the effect of three nights of selective slow-wave sleep suppression in young healthy subjects and found that participants became less sensitive to insulin, resulting in reduced tolerance to glucose and increased risk for Type 2 diabetes. Riva *et al.* (2010) found that women with fibromyalgia syndrome had less sleep and impaired quality of sleep compared with a matched group of healthy women. Individuals sleeping well, on the other hand, seem to be more resistant to stress-related disorders, even when exposed to intense and long-term stress.

ALLOSTATIC LOAD

The Allostatic Load model of McEwen (1998) describes the conditions under which bodily responses to stress are health promoting rather than health damaging. Allostasis refers to the ability of the body to reach stability through change. Certain bodily systems, such as body temperature and blood carbon dioxide level, have to be kept stable whereas other systems, such as blood pressure and heart rate, can vary substantially to meet environmental demands. According to the Allostatic Load model (Fig. 5.4), a normal healthy response to stress involves the rapid activation of bodily systems, which helps the individual to cope with the stressor. However, it is equally important to be able to shut off these responses as soon as the stress is over. The mobilisation of energy through catabolic mechanisms has to be balanced by anabolic processes in order to accumulate resources for future demands and contribute to growth, regeneration, healing, digestion and reproduction. The physiological stress responses, which at first can be supportive of coping, may when they are prolonged cause damage to the body. The frequent or chronic activation of the allostatic systems, with too little or no time at all for rest and recovery, will increase the wear and tear of the organism and may, for example, cause the dysregulation of bodily systems and inability to cope adequately with new demands. Also an inadequate (blunted) response may cause health problems by not mobilising necessary coping resources. Inability to mobilise resources by one system may also cause compensatory overactivation of other systems. For example, inability to activate the HPA axis in response to stress (hypocortisolism) may cause overactivity of the immune system with inflammatory responses, allergies, oversensitivity, rheumatism and eczema.

Thus, from a long-term health perspective, a reasonable balance is necessary between activation and rest/recovery. Overexposure to stress responses can be caused by unremitting stress. In laboratory experiments with monkeys, Jay Kaplan and his group (2009) at Bowman Gray University in the USA have exposed the animals to chronic social stress by repeatedly introducing unacquainted monkeys into the group. This causes social disruption and stress in the animals when they try to establish a new social rank order. This process was associated with elevation in blood pressure and increased speed of atherosclerosis, thus increasing the risk of heart attacks, compared with monkeys with the same food and physical environment but not exposed to psychosocial stress. Similar processes are likely to occur in employees

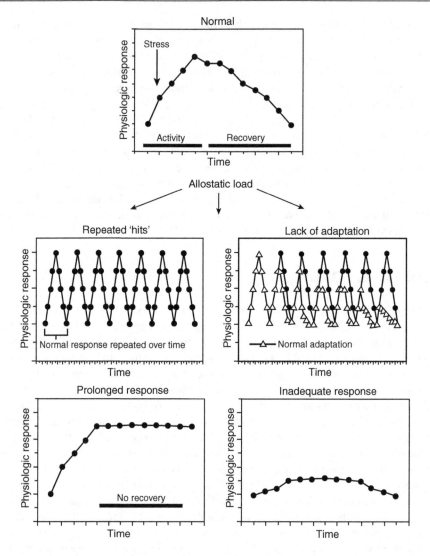

Fig. 5.4 Allostatic load. Reprinted from McEwen (1998) with permission.

who are exposed to frequent reorganisations that require them to adjust to new conditions and new colleagues repeatedly, leading to their social position being undermined and unclear.

The increase in health problems in Eastern Europe and the reduction in life expectancy in men in Russia after the collapse of Communism in 1989 are examples of negative health outcomes assumed to be caused by major social, economic and political changes in these countries. These processes started rather suddenly, but the consequences in terms of elevated psychosocial stress exposure are long-lasting as the economic, political and social turbulence is still considerable. As pointed out above, stress-related health problems in the new EU member states, most of them once part of the former Soviet Union, are much more widespread than in the rest of EU.

Chronic stress is thus known to take its toll in many ways, contributing to cardiovascular disorders, impairment of the immune system, diabetes and other chronic illnesses.

Frequently repeated mental stress exposure may cause similar problems. If blood pressure and heart rate are activated too often without adequate physical output, blood vessels in the coronary arteries are damaged and clogged, which speeds up the atherosclerotic process leading to heart attacks. CHD mortality is four times higher in 50-year-old Lithuanian men than in 50-year-old Swedish men (Kristenson, 1998). This difference cannot be explained by standard risk factors. Kristenson examined differences in psychosocial risk factors for CHD in the two countries and found that men from Vilnius, Lithuania, compared with those from Linköping, Sweden, had higher job strain, lower social and emotional support at work, higher vital exhaustion and depression and lower coping resources, self-esteem, social integration and sense of coherence. Vilnius men also showed a lower quality of working life and perceived health. Kristenson *et al.* (1998) also investigated cortisol reactivity to a standardised laboratory stress test in population-based random samples of 50-year-old men from Vilnius and Linköping, and found a low peak cortisol response in men from Vilnius, which was significantly related to high baseline cortisol, current smoking, and vital exhaustion. The findings suggest that chronic psychosocial stress in Vilnius men is related to elevated baseline cortisol and an attenuated response to challenge. According to the Allostatic Load model, this is likely to represent an example of an inadequate stress response, which is likely to be caused by long-term exposure to stressful conditions.

A measure of allostatic load can be calculated as the combined effect on a number of physiological systems such as heart rate, blood lipids, glucose metabolism, stress hormones, etc. (McEwen, 1998; Evans, 2003; Lindfors *et al.*, 2006). Even if single biomarkers do not exceed traditional risk levels, the cumulative load of a number of biological systems being strained may cause health problems. Sleep disturbance and insufficient relaxation are associated with elevated cortisol levels (Ekstedt *et al.*, 2004; Gustafsson *et al.*, 2008). Stress-induced sleep disturbance and lack of restitution may start a vicious circle in which the individual has to mobilise extra resources each morning to be able to cope with daily hassles. At first this will help the individual to cope with daily stress and demands despite insufficient rest, but if this condition continues regulatory mechanisms are disturbed and dysregulation may occur. This can be seen in terms of over- as well as under-activity of bodily processes. Whereas acute stress causes an increase in cortisol secretion, long-term exposure to stress results in a disruption of central regulatory systems and a decrease in cortisol output.

Patients with post-traumatic stress disorder (PTSD), chronic fatigue syndrome (CFS), fibromyalgia and burnout syndromes or similar disorders may sometimes be hypersensitive and sometimes apathetic. In a population-based case-control study of 83 individuals suffering from CFS, Maloney *et al.* (2009) found that persons with CFS were significantly more likely to have a high allostatic load based on 11 biomarkers: heart rate, systolic and diastolic blood pressure, waist/hip ratio, HDL and total cholesterol, glucose, insulin, C-reactive protein, albumin and salivary cortisol. Following a review of available evidence on CFS and HPA axis function, Van Houdenhove *et al.* (2009) concluded that CFS is characterised by hypocortisolism (low cortisol levels) and represents a persistent dysregulation of the neurobiological stress systems. The balance between HPA axis activity and inflammatory responses is disturbed, and enhanced inflammatory activity releases cytokines. This affects the brain and provokes feelings of sickness reflected in low-grade fever, sensory hypersensitivity, low mood, sleepiness, concentration problems and social withdrawal.

Another condition assumed to be caused by chronic stress is fibromyalgia syndrome (FMS) (Kivimäki *et al.*, 2004). Patients suffering from FMS characteristically have widespread musculoskeletal pain and diffuse tenderness, and can be diagnosed on the basis of a number of pain trigger points. Fibromyalgia patients present lower pain thresholds and report higher pain ratings in response to different stimuli (Granges & Littlejohn, 1993; Desmeules *et al.*, 2003; Petzke *et al.*, 2003). A possible explanation is structural changes in the pain system. In addition, fibromyalgia patients display a number of somatic and psychological symptoms and report more stress than matched controls (Riva *et al.*, 2010). In addition, their stress systems are often dysregulated. Wingenfeld *et al.* (2007) compared fibromyalgia patients with a matched group of patients with pelvic pain and healthy controls and found that the group with fibromyalgia showed an attenuated cortisol response when exposed to experimental stress compared with the other groups. Crofford *et al.* (2004) found that fibromyalgia patients had elevated cortisol levels in the evening compared with a control group. Riva *et al.* (2010) compared 29 female fibromyalgia patients with 29 matched healthy controls in terms of cortisol on waking and during the day and found that the patients had significantly lower cortisol, especially on waking and during the following hour, i.e. an attenuated cortisol awakening response (CAR). This indicates that these patients are unable to mobilise necessary resources for starting and fulfilling a day at work. This is consistent with their feelings of lack of energy and chronic fatigue. However, it is unclear whether fibromyalgia is caused by the dysregulation of the cortisol system (hypocortisolism) or if dysregulation is caused by fibromyalgia. Heart rate in these patients was elevated compared with a matched group of healthy women (Riva *et al.*, 2010), and this difference was most pronounced during non-stressful and relaxing conditions. This could indicate a compensatory response of the sympathetic nervous system in which the response of the HPA axis is attenuated, or illustrate a general dysfunction of the regulation of the physiological stress responses (over- as well as underactivity).

FMS patients have been found to display under-, over-, as well as normal, activity of the HPA axis (Catley *et al.*, 2000, and others). In addition to possible methodological differences between studies, a likely explanation for the contradictory results (over- as well as underactivity) is that chronic stress first leads to hyperactivity of the HPA axis, followed by dysregulation of this system and a successive decline in the response, ending up in underactivity (Rosmond & Björntorp, 2000; Miller *et al.*, 2007; Van Houdenhove *et al.*, 2009). Depending on the duration of stress exposure and individual differences in coping abilities, seemingly contradictory results can be explained. This is very much in line with Selye's classical three-stage General Adaptation Syndrome (Selye, 1956). The first response to stress in terms of novelty or threat is the 'alarm reaction', which is followed by 'recovery' if the stress situation is over, or 'resistance' if stress continues. During the 'resistance stage' the organism repairs itself and stores energy. If stress becomes overwhelming or prolonged, exhaustion sets in and may eventually lead to breakdown and death of the organism. Selye's work was based on animal research but human examples of the third stage of his model can be found in terms of vital exhaustion, apathy, burnout, chronic fatigue syndromes and *karoshi* deaths.

A phenomenon named 'apathetic children' has received great attention and concern, and started a debate in Sweden in recent years. An 'epidemic' of apathetic children started in 2005 among children of refugees from countries with ongoing war, armed conflicts between different ethnic and/or religious groups and groups exposed to persecution and with an unsecure future. These children lie in bed without eating or communicating. They are kept alive with tube-feeding in hospitals, and their parents are unable to give them trust and security as they themselves are in a stressful and uncontrollable situation. Many refugees have been waiting a long time for asylum or have already been informed that the family will be expelled. In some cases one or both parents are dead. The state of these children is very similar to the stage of exhaustion described by Selye, and their social situation is characterised by severe chronic stress without any control or coping resources. From an evolutionary perspective, this condition can be compared to the 'playing dead' response found in some animals. Sharks, lizards, snakes and spiders can place themselves in a tonic immobility state. This is likely to play a role in survival of animals as a hunted, inanimate 'playing dead' animal may be difficult to spot and some predators only catch live prey. Also rodents and birds can stay immobile when a predator is approaching, but rapidly switch to activation and run or fly away when the threat is too close. Through evolution and a common origin, similarities can easily be found in different species of animals and in humans as ways of coping with threatening situations such as uncontrollable stress. However, what is adaptive in some species and in some situations may be maladaptive for others. 'Apathetic children' would not survive unless treated in hospital. In cases where the family's social situation improved, most children recovered.

Work-related risk factors, certain individual characteristics and unhealthy lifestyles are factors assumed to contribute to increased allostatic load. Alavinia *et al.* (2009) evaluated the relative contribution of individual characteristics, lifestyle factors, work-related risk factors and work ability to sickness absence in 5867 Dutch construction workers. Work-related factors included questionnaire measures of physical load and psychosocial characteristics of the job, according to Karasek's Job Content Questionnaire. After adjusting for the effects of work ability on sickness absence, individual factors such as obesity, smoking and work-related factors such as manual materials handling and lack of job control were important predictors of long durations of sick leave. It was concluded that interventions to reduce smoking, obesity, physical load, psychosocial work factors and gaining control over the job would be the most efficient means of reducing sick leave.

CATABOLIC AND ANABOLIC PROCESSES

Activation of bodily systems, which is usually initiated by signals from the hypothalamus and the sympathetic nervous system and the production of stress hormones such as adrenaline, noradrenaline and cortisol, means that resources in the body are mobilised for active coping and 'fight or flight'. This 'catabolic process' is of importance for survival and protection of the body. However, these resources have to be regenerated and restored. Chronic activation will deplete these resources, induce imbalance between different physiological systems and processes and disturb regulatory mechanisms, which can cause over- as well as under-reactivity to external stimuli. Inadequate functioning of these systems will reduce the individual's ability to cope with new demands.

In contrast to the catabolic processes involved in activity, conditions such as rest, recovery and sleep induce anabolic processes stimulated by the secretion of anabolic hormones such as the sex hormones (oestrogen, testosterone) and growth hormones. Since the hypothalamus regulates both stress responses and the sex hormones, it is easy to understand how stress can influence the production of oestrogen and testosterone. The anabolic processes involve storage of energy via metabolic activity, growth, regeneration, healing, repair, reproduction and improved immune functions. Deep slow-wave sleep is of particular importance for anabolic processes, and sleep is also of importance for memory consolidation. Moderate regular physical activity and pleasant stimulation (e.g. music and singing) are also factors that contribute to reduce stress and activate anabolic processes.

During active work the secretion of stress hormones is increased whereas the production of sex and growth hormones is reduced. Under stressful conditions, digestion and healing processes slow down and sexual desire and reproductive functions are suppressed. As a consequence, women under severe stress may stop menstruating, and menstruation may become irregular under chronic stress exposure. Examples of this can be found among women athletes undergoing excessive physical training, such as female marathon runners, who develop anovulation, irregular menstrual cycles and 'runner's amenorrhoea'. In young girls severe mental or physical stress may prevent and postpone their first menstrual bleed (menarche). Their bodies do not develop breasts, or accumulate fat on hips and thighs, until they reduce their training and stress. Stress can affect infertility both by the altered regulation of pituitary hormones and from nervous-system influences on the ovaries. Elias *et al.* (2005) assessed the effect of childhood exposure to the 1944–1945 Dutch famine on subsequent female reproductive function and found a longstanding but modest effect of childhood famine exposure on reproductive function in women. In men, extreme stress can reduce sperm count. From an evolutionary perspective, this seems logical as having children under conditions characterised by severe long-term stress is not optimal for survival.

For long-term health a reasonable balance is necessary between catabolic and anabolic processes, that is, between activity and rest/recovery. Humans can be exposed to relatively intense and long-term stress without noticeable health problems, but sooner or later there must be opportunities for rest and recovery to restore important functions and regenerate depleted resources. However, there are considerable individual differences in susceptibility to stress depending on earlier experiences, genetic factors, and social, emotional and material coping resources and strategies. Vulnerable individuals may develop symptoms relatively rapidly compared with more resistant individuals. In a stressful job it may take years to develop serious stress-related symptoms for some individuals, whereas others may develop similar symptoms within months.

6 Stress-related Health Problems

Relationships between occupational and other forms of stress and health outcomes have been demonstrated in a great number of studies. Several links between occupational stress and health have already been described in previous chapters. The aim of this chapter is to summarise scientific evidence for the possible psychobiological mechanisms involved in some of these relationships. Learning about these mechanisms is important for prevention as well as for treatment of stress-related disorders. Biomarkers of these processes can also be used as warning signals in potentially stressful work situations, and as outcome measures in response to interventions to promote health in working life. Through a better understanding of the underlying mechanisms of stress-related disorders, patients suffering from such health problems are recognised as 'real' patients and their symptoms are taken more seriously. Many patients suffering from diffuse pain symptoms, sleeping problems and depression feel that they are to blame themselves, and that their problems are all in their head (imagined). As many of them have sought medical help repeatedly without receiving any diagnosis and, consequently, no effective treatment has been offered, they feel helpless and expect their condition to continue or get worse, which eventually results in feelings of hopelessness and chronic disease.

As stress may cause dysregulation of central systems in the body, it is not surprising that stress-related symptoms may appear in many different forms, mental as well as physical. Kudielka *et al.* (2006) performed a review of the empirical evidence for a dysregulation of the HPA axis in chronic stress conditions such as burnout and vital exhaustion, concluding that chronic stress seems to be associated with dysregulation of basal cortisol secretion and cortisol reactivity under stress, but that the direction of change is inconsistent. Depending on individual differences in genetic factors (including sex), early experiences and present situation, symptoms may vary considerably between individuals exposed to the same occupational situation. However, some stress-related disorders are more common than others. As mentioned earlier, muscular pain, chronic fatigue, depression, burnout syndromes, sleep disturbances, memory problems and feeling stressed are the most frequently reported health problems among workers in the European Union. In Sweden, for instance, about 50% of sickness absenteeism is due to psychological problems, of which depression constitutes 35%. MSD is the second most common reason for absenteeism from work, with psychosocial stress likely to play an important role for the development and maintenance of these problems.

The Science of Occupational Health: Stress, Psychobiology and the New World of Work, first edition
By Ulf Lundberg and Cary L. Cooper. Published 2011 by Blackwell Publishing Ltd
© 2011 Ulf Lundberg and Cary L. Cooper

CHRONIC FATIGUE, DEPRESSION, BURNOUT

Conditions such as chronic fatigue, depression, burnout and fibromyalgia are considered to be associated with dysregulation of the HPA axis in terms of over- or underproduction of cortisol. A greater understanding of the mechanisms linking cortisol secretion to various health conditions has been obtained in recent years, thanks to researchers in the USA such as Robert Sapolsky at Stanford University and Bruce McEwen at Rockefeller University. Conditions such as Cushing's syndrome, depression, Type 2 diabetes and sleep deprivation are usually associated with overproduction of cortisol, whereas chronic fatigue syndrome, fibromyalgia, allergies and rheumatoid arthritis are linked to underproduction. Chronically elevated cortisol levels can be induced by intensive mental stress and by excessive physical exercise, causing weight loss, lack of menstruation, anorexia and insulin resistance. Insulin resistance is a risk factor for Type 2 or non-insulin-dependent diabetes.

Patients with Cushing's syndrome illustrate some of the effects of an overproduction of cortisol (hypercortisolism). This syndrome is usually caused by a tumour in the pituitary, stimulating the production of ACTH to induce very high cortisol secretion from the adrenals. Patients with Cushing's syndrome are characterised by depression, memory impairment, high susceptibility to infections and accumulation of fat in the abdominal region, and elevated risk of developing CVD and Type 2 diabetes. Memory impairment is related to the effects of chronically elevated cortisol levels on the hippocampus. Hippocampal atrophy has also been found in individuals exposed to long-lasting traumatic stress (e.g. PTSD). Chronic stress exposure induces similar effects (Fig. 6.1).

An association between cortisol and depression has been known for a long time (Sachar & Baron, 1979). High baseline levels of cortisol are assumed to increase the risk of depression,

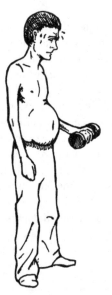

• Abdominal fat accumulation

• Reduced reproductive activity (sex and growth hormones)

• Cardiovascular disease (elevated free fatty acids, atherosclerosis, blood clotting)

• Infections, slow healing (impaired immune function)

• Type 2 diabetes (insulin resistance)

• Memory impairment (degeneration of hippocampus)

Fig. 6.1   Health problems associated with dysregulation of the HPA axis and high cortisol levels. Drawing by Urban Skytt.

but depression is also likely to influence cortisol levels. Patients with depression tend to have a 'flatter' cortisol curve over the day, with relatively low morning and relatively high afternoon and evening values. Lack of cortisol in the morning (attenuated cortisol awakening response) will cause lack of energy, which makes it difficult to get out of bed and perform daily activities such as going to work and doing a proper job. Elevated cortisol levels in the evening may interfere with food intake and digestion (no appetite, stomach problems) and sleep (difficulties falling asleep, reduced slow-wave sleep, frequent waking up during the night). In this way, depression usually also leads to the development of various physical symptoms. Furthermore, research generally shows that depression is independently associated with increased cardiovascular morbidity and mortality (Lichtman et al., 2008).

However, the relation between depression, stress and cortisol secretion is complex. Peeters et al. (2003) investigated cortisol responses to daily events and found blunted responses in patients with major depressive disorder compared with healthy controls. Preussner et al. (2003) found that higher levels of self-reported depressive symptomatology in 40 healthy men were associated with a greater cortisol response after awakening. Preussner et al. (1999) also investigated cortisol responses in male and female teachers and found differential effects of burnout (lower cortisol) and perceived stress (increased cortisol levels). In a study comparing 22 postmenopausal depressed women with 23 age-matched healthy women, Weber-Hamann et al. (2002) found that hypercortisolaemic depressed patients had greater insulin resistance and increased visceral fat. Everson-Rose et al. (2009) examined the association between depressive symptoms and abdominal (visceral) fat and subcutaneous fat, respectively, in 409 middle-aged women. Visceral fat constitutes a greater cardiovascular risk than subcutaneous fat. Women with clinically relevant depressive scores had about 35% more visceral fat compared with women with lower scores, but no association was found with subcutaneous fat. It was concluded that visceral fat may be one pathway between depression and CVD. Mason et al. (2002) investigated combat veterans with post-traumatic stress disorder and concluded that there was a central regulatory dysfunction of the HPA axis in PTSD patients who showed a dynamic tendency to overreact with hyper- or hypocortisolism to psychosocial stress. In conclusion, dysregulation of the HPA axis may cause suppressed as well as enhanced cortisol secretion.

Severe stressful events, such as exposure to war, rape and torture, may lead to serious stress-related disorders within days or weeks. Under more 'normal' work-related stress, the development of such serious health problems usually takes months or years. In view of this, it should not be a surprise that it also usually takes a long time, often years, to recover from such disorders, even with proper treatment. Treatment of burnout syndrome and similar conditions can be successful, making it possible for the patient to recover and return to work. However, even after recovery, there seem to be lasting effects in terms of increased stress sensitivity. After return to work, people have to be particularly careful not to be exposed to severe stress, and to make sure that they have enough time for rest, recovery, recuperation and relaxing activities, including regular physical exercise. Usually work tasks and work organisation have to be adjusted to the employee's new situation. Workers who after treatment return to the same work situation that caused their stress problems often rapidly develop the same symptoms again. The body seems to have learned that this is a harmful situation and responds rapidly with symptoms. It is likely that central bodily functions have altered their sensitivity to stressful stimuli. Under non-stressful conditions, an individual who has been treated for PTSD or burnout may seem healthy and may carry out daily chores and their job in a normal way. However, if exposed to stressful conditions, he or she seems to be more vulnerable than before and responds with excessive stress reactions and, eventually, develops the same condition as before. Individuals who develop these disorders in the first place may often have been exposed to traumatic events as a child. For example, abuse and violence, drugs, death in the family, divorce and parental conflicts are events that are more common among patients with burnout syndrome. Experiences early in life seem to have a strong influence on the development and regulation of children's stress systems, and may also make them more vulnerable to stress as adults. This 'programming' of the stress systems is very much in line with results from animal experiments by Meaney and his colleagues on the effects of treatment of rat pups on their stress responses as adults, described in Chapter 5.

CARDIOVASCULAR DISORDERS

Serious cardiovascular disease (CVD), principally myocardial infarction and stroke, is not as common in the working population (compared with other health problems), but represents the most common reason for death in the Western world. About 50% of the population die from CVD. This has created an interest in factors contributing to CVD, and stress has for a long time been considered to be of importance. For people contracting CVD at an early age, work conditions are assumed to play an important role. In a recent systematic review by Eller *et al.* (2009), evidence was found for an association between work-related psychosocial factors (high psychological demands; lack of social support; iso-strain, i.e. the combination of low control and high demands at work) and ischaemic heart disease. Furthermore, psychosocial and physical conditions at work contribute to the development of risk factors resulting in heart attacks and stroke later in life. As mentioned earlier, important risk factors for heart attack, in addition to stress, are smoking, high blood pressure, diabetes, lack of exercise, unhealthy diet and overweight; and many of these factors are also related to workplace stress. The mechanisms linking psychosocial stress and behaviour to CVD, such as myocardial infarction, have been investigated extensively. In addition to the indirect effects of stress on lifestyle, the following series of events has been suggested and supported by animal models (Fig. 6.2):

1. Psychosocial stress causes an increase in blood pressure and heart rate as well as a release of energy in terms of glucose and free fatty acids into the blood stream.

Atherosclerosis

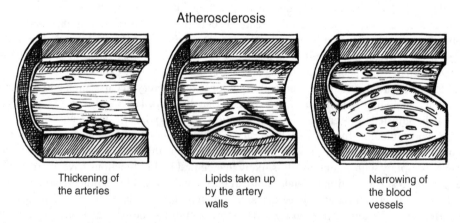

| Thickening of the arteries | Lipids taken up by the artery walls | Narrowing of the blood vessels |

Fig. 6.2 Stress contributes to atherosclerosis and blood clotting. Drawing by Urban Skytt.

2. Frequent or chronic elevation of the blood pressure contributes to structural changes in the arteries, for example in the coronary arteries supplying blood to the heart itself (the myocardium).
3. Long-term exposure to high blood pressure and/or repeated elevation of blood pressure lead to thicker and stiffer walls of the blood vessels and a smaller diameter (lumen), which increases vascular resistance and reduces blood flow. Increased resistance causes increased blood pressure (diastolic blood pressure in particular), but also a compensatory increase in systolic blood pressure to transport oxygen and nutrients more efficiently through the narrow vessels to the muscle cells of the heart.
4. A high heart rate and elevated blood pressure may cause damage to the inner walls (endothelium) of the blood vessels, particularly where a vessel branches off.
5. Fatty acids will be built into the walls at these places in the blood vessels and form foam cells in the intima (atherosclerosis).
6. The high level of blood lipids during stress will enhance the atherosclerotic process.
7. A narrowing of the coronary arteries due to thicker walls and atherosclerosis will reduce the blood flow to the myocardium. The individual will experience chest pain (angina) when exposed to physical and mental effort requiring more energy and oxygen than is supplied to the heart.
8. Blood clotting (coagulation) increases during stress and will in combination with atherosclerosis further increase the risk of a myocardial infarction, i.e. a complete obstruction of the blood flow to parts of the heart muscle.
9. Furthermore, atherosclerotic arteries have been found to respond paradoxically to stressful demands by vasoconstriction rather than by vasodilation (Harris & Matthews, 2004).

IMMUNE FUNCTION

In an acute stress situation, the immune system is activated and immune cells move to sites where they are needed. This has an important protective function which reduces the effects of injuries and infections. Chronically elevated cortisol levels, however, have an immunosup-pressive effect. An impairment of the immune system means that the individual becomes more susceptible to infections. Invasion of the body by viruses or bacteria is not sufficient to cause a disease. The role of the immune system is to identify and attack these pathogens. If the immune system is compromised, the risk of an infection increases after exposure to the disease-causing agent. The relation between stress and susceptibility to the common cold has been demonstrated experimentally in a series of studies by Sheldon Cohen and his colleagues (Cohen, 2005), at Carnegie Mellon University in Pittsburgh, USA. The common cold is very prevalent. Adults have on average about two to four colds per year, and smokers and individuals with low socioeconomic status are at an increased risk of contracting the common cold. It causes a lot of workplace sickness absence and the economic impact of the common cold is enormous, estimated in the USA to exceed $20 billion annually. Reducing the number of colds would thus have extensive positive economic benefits. In the USA, colds occur most commonly from late August to early April, but, contrary to widespread belief, being chilled and damp does not increase susceptibility to the common cold. Colds are more common in the winter months because that is when people are more likely to be indoors, which facilitates the spread of viruses. The immune system has an important role also in healing processes, and evidence is accumulating that shows that these processes slow down during chronic stress.

Janice Kiecolt-Glaser and her colleagues at Ohio State University, USA, have performed a number of experiments on stress and healing processes, and have shown that stress reduction speeds up healing (Kiecolt-Glaser *et al.*, 1995). This is of considerable importance, for example in surgery, by reducing costs incurred through hospitalisation. In addition, through faster healing the risk of infections is reduced and patients recover from pain more rapidly.

Cohen's experimental model, tested at the Common Cold Unit of the Medical Research Council in Salisbury, UK, consists of comparing healthy individuals, exposed to different levels of stress, in terms of their susceptibility to the common cold virus (rhinovirus). Nasal drops containing a rhinovirus are administered to healthy participants, who are then kept under strict control in the laboratory for a few days. During this period objective signs of infection are recorded (coughing, a runny nose, etc.) and verified by analysing antibodies to the rhinovirus. About 35% of all participants exposed to the virus developed signs of having a common cold (coughing, excessive mucus production, etc.), but differences in prevalence were related to the amount of previous stress exposure. For example, individuals exposed to two years of stress were found to be four times as likely to become infected compared with individuals not exposed to stress at all, after controlling for possible confounders (Fig. 6.3; Cohen *et al.*, 1998). Similarly, he has demonstrated increased susceptibility to the common cold in individuals with low SES and low social support. In summary, his experiments consistently show a strong graded relation between the amount of stress exposure and the risk of becoming infected. Lower risk for developing a cold has been found among individuals with positive emotional style and a greater number of social roles (Cohen *et al.*, 2003). It is likely, that similar relations exist for other infections. Latent viruses, such as herpes, are known to flare up under conditions characterised by mental and physical stress. As mentioned above, Cohen *et al.* (2009) also found that amount and quality of sleep was related to susceptibility to the common cold.

Individual biological responses (cortisol, adrenaline, noradrenaline, blood pressure, heart rate) to acute stressors are relatively constant and hence represent a stable individual trait. The magnitude of the cortisol response to acute stress is of particular interest, as cortisol can suppress the inflammatory immune response. A greater release of cortisol in an acute stress situation could thus be associated with greater susceptibility to infections under chronic

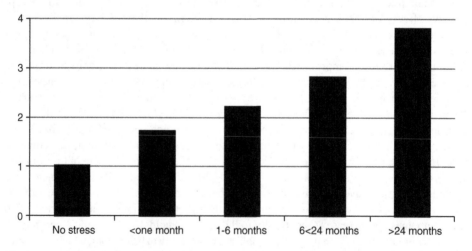

Fig. 6.3   Relative risk of developing common cold as related to the duration of stress. Based on Cohen *et al.* (1998) with permission.

stress. Cohen *et al.* (2002) investigated the relation between high versus low cortisol reactivity to acute experimental stress and high levels of stressful life events earlier in life, and the incidence of upper respiratory illness (verified colds) in 115 healthy subjects followed during 12 weeks in their natural settings. Participants with a high amount of negative life events experienced a higher number of verified cold episodes than participants with low levels of negative life events, but the difference was most pronounced for individuals who were high in cortisol reactivity. Among participants with a high cortisol response to experimental stress (preparation and delivery of a laboratory speech task), almost 60% of those with a high amount of negative life events experienced a verified cold episode compared with less than 10% among those with a low amount of negative life events. The corresponding difference among participants with a low cortisol response to experimental stress was much smaller, about 20% versus 10% with verified colds. Immune responses to the laboratory stress were consistent with the cortisol responses and show that laboratory markers reflect individual vulnerability to increased risk of upper respiratory illness in the natural environment.

A possible mechanism through which stress may increase vulnerability to infectious disease is a poorer antibody response. This was demonstrated by Miller *et al.* (2004) who administered an influenza vaccine to young adults reporting different levels of stress. The reduced antibody response was found to be most pronounced about 10 days after increased stress.

Experiments on healing processes show that it takes much longer for wounds to heal when the individual has been under stress. Kiecolt-Glaser *et al.* (1995) investigated the effects of stress on wound healing in 13 women caring for a relative with Alzheimer's disease, compared with 13 controls matched for age and family income. All subjects underwent a 3.5-mm punch biopsy wound. It was found that wound healing took significantly longer in caregivers than in controls (48 compared with 39 days). In another study from this group (Marucha *et al.*, 1998), wounds experimentally induced in students were found to take about 40% longer to heal during examination periods compared with vacation time. The clinical application of this finding was investigated in a study by Broadbent *et al.* (2003). Forty-seven adult patients were asked to assess their psychological stress and worry using a standardised questionnaire before undergoing surgery. It was found that high levels of stress and worry were associated with impaired wound repair following surgery. This finding suggests that, in clinical practice, interventions to reduce stress can improve the speed of healing and shorten length and costs of hospital stay.

COGNITIVE FUNCTION

Cortisol enters the brain. In this way the brain can monitor and regulate cortisol levels in blood and send signals to increase or decrease secretion from the adrenals depending on internal and external demands. Normal levels promote the storage of memory but chronically high cortisol levels can impair memory functions (Sapolsky, 1996; McEwen & Lasley, 2002). The hippocampal formation, which is an area of the brain of importance for memory and other cognitive functions such as spatial navigation, seems to be particularly sensitive. High cortisol levels enter the brain and cause hippocampal atrophy. The connections (dendrites) between brain cells (neurons) are destroyed, and cortisol also promotes loss of nerve cells. This is reflected in reduced hippocampal volume and impaired memory function and spatial navigation. Patients with Cushing's syndrome, people with PTSD from combat, children exposed to sexual abuse and people who have suffered from depression tend to have smaller hippocampi than healthy individuals and also display memory problems. The longer people have suffered from depression, the smaller their hippocampus. Starkman *et al.* (1992) showed that the reduction in volume of this area and the loss of memory are proportional to the amount of cortisol secreted. Starkman *et al.* (2001) also compared 48 patients with Cushing's disease and 38 healthy controls in terms of cortisol levels and cognitive performance (IQ test) and found that verbal learning was significantly decreased among patients with the disease.

Fortunately, the stress-induced atrophy of the hippocampus is reversible. If stress and cortisol levels are reduced, the connections between neurons are re-established and memory functions are improved, as demonstrated in a longitudinal study of elderly women by Seeman *et al.* (1997). Women who reduced their cortisol levels over the years improved their memory and increased the volume of the hippocampus, whereas women who increased their cortisol levels showed the opposite.

Chronic stress is also assumed to cause death of neurons. However, the importance of this is not quite clear as the brain is rather plastic and can lose a number of cells without obvious behavioural, cognitive and emotional symptoms. In addition, new neurons are produced in the hippocampal formation and regular moderate physical activity and pleasant experiences seem to contribute to this production. Hippocampus is one of very few brain regions where new neurons are created throughout life (Kuruba *et al.*, 2009). In an experimental study (Bendel *et al.*, 2005), rats were exposed to global brain ischaemia (reduced oxygen supply), which caused neural death in the hippocampus and impaired learning and memory. However, during the following months, new brain cells were produced in this area, and three months after the ischaemia learning and memory functions had returned to normal. These results show that the brain has the capacity to form new nerve cells after injury and that this contributes to a restoration of cognitive functions of the brain. The creation of new neurons has been found to be influenced by lifestyle factors, such as physical activity and a stimulating life. Regular moderate but not excessive physical exercise has been shown to significantly enhance the formation of new brain cells in the hippocampus. Increased cortisol levels and chronic stress can suppress the production of new cells, whereas animal experiments (Kemperman *et al.*, 1997) have shown that an enriched environment can increase the production of new cells. Naylor *et al.* (2005) examined the effects of different amounts of voluntary running in rats and found that a moderate amount of running was beneficial for the formation of new brain cells in the hippocampus, whereas long periods of excessive voluntary running were associated with physiological stress responses and an inhibition of exercise-induced formation of new brain cells. Lack of physical activity also reduced the formation of new brain cells in the hippocampus in the rats. The implications for those at work in high-pressure jobs is obvious. It is important to stay active, to engage in physical exercise and to be involved in stimulating work and non-work activities.

OBESITY, DIABETES — THE METABOLIC SYNDROME

The fat depot in the central part of the body is a source of energy that can be useful under certain chronic stressful conditions, such as when exposed to high physical demands or lack of nutrition. The fat in this region is readily released into the body in terms of free fatty acids, which gives energy to the cells. However, if this energy is not needed for physical activity and if food supply is normal (or excessive), elevated lipid levels will contribute to atherosclerosis and cardiovascular disorders.

High cortisol levels contribute to insulin resistance. Compared with Type 1 diabetes, which is due to inability to produce insulin because the insulin-producing cells in the pancreas have been destroyed by the immune system, Type 2 diabetes is characterised by normal or even elevated insulin levels. However, the uptake of glucose by the cells from the blood is reduced because of the insensitivity to insulin caused by high cortisol levels. Chronic stress and high cortisol levels, abdominal fat accumulation, high blood lipids and blood pressure, together with Type 2 diabetes, form the dominating part of the 'metabolic syndrome', which is an important risk factor for cardiovascular disease. Measures of waist–hip ratio or waist circumference are more sensitive indicators of the metabolic syndrome and cardiovascular risk than the traditional body mass index (weight divided by height in square metres). Balkau *et al.* (2007) investigated waist circumference and body mass index (BMI) as risk factors for CVD and diabetes in 63 countries with about 170 000 patients aged 18 to 80 in the International Day for the Evaluation of Abdominal Obesity (IDEA) study. A statistically significant graded increase existed in the frequency of CVD and diabetes mellitus with both BMI and waist circumference, with a stronger relationship with waist circumference than with BMI for both genders. According to a Swedish study with 2077 patients, also part of the IDEA study (Wittchen *et al.*, 2006), 47% of men and 52% of women with a waist circumference greater than 101 cm had hypertension, and 24% and 28% respectively had diabetes. A strong association between abdominal fat and social conditions was found. Men and women on sick leave had higher waist circumference than working and unemployed individuals, but men and women with university education had lower. It was also found that smokers and ex-smokers had higher waist circumference than non-smokers, and that people living in cities had lower waist circumference than people in rural areas. Similarly, Sjöholm (2007) found that waist circumference was a stronger predictor of hypertension than BMI. For example, for men with a waist circumference of more than 100 cm, the risk of hypertension was almost 10 times greater than for men with a waist circumference less than 80 cm. In conclusion, waist circumference is a relevant measure of abdominal fat accumulation and more strongly related to the development of hypertension than the traditional BMI measure of overweight.

With stress, overweight and obesity increasing problems in a large part of the working world, Type 2 diabetes has increased dramatically and is expected to increase further. For example, in the USA almost 30% of the population is obese (body mass index >30). Certain ethnic groups that have undergone rapid changes from conditions characterised by lack of nutrition to a condition with easy access to unlimited amounts of (fast) high-fat and carbohydrate-rich food have shown a rapid increase in obesity and Type 2 diabetes. Typical examples are aborigines in Australia, some native Indian tribes in USA, and Inuits in Greenland. Also people from India moving to UK have shown a similar pattern with increased abdominal fat. An extreme example is the small republic of Nauru in the South Pacific. Until the 1970s, Nauruans used to live a physically active life and ate a low-fat diet of fish and native fruit and vegetables. Then it became one of the wealthiest countries in the world from phosphate mining. This new-found wealth was followed by extensive lifestyle changes and increased workplace stress. Nauru came to possess one of the highest rates of diabetes in the world. In 1975, the overall prevalence of diabetes was 34.4% and a further 11.3% were at high risk of developing diabetes. Two-thirds of the population aged 15 years and over were smokers, 73% of these smoking more than 20 cigarettes per day, and 26% smoking more than 40 per day. Nauru also has the highest rates of obesity in the world, 80% having a BMI greater than 30.

MUSCULOSKELETAL DISORDERS

Musculoskeletal disorders (MSD) such as neck, shoulder and back pain problems are one of the most widespread occupational diseases. According to the European Agency for Safety and Health at Work (2008), 25% of workers in the 27 EU countries report suffering from backache and 23% complain of muscular pains. The total costs of back pain in the OECD countries have been estimated at 1–2% of the gross national product (Nordlund & Waddell, 2000) as a result of loss of productivity and sickness absence. Silverstein and Adams (2007) found that neck, back and upper extremity work-related MSDs represent 27% of all workers' compensation claims in the state of Washington, USA.

For a long time these disorders were linked mainly to physical work conditions. Heavy lifting and bad ergonomic conditions, such as twisting the body and lifting at the same time, and working with arms above the shoulders, as well as repetitive physical movements or static load, are important risk factors for MSD (Bernard, 1997). Technical improvements in the industrialised countries in terms of more use of lifting cranes and trucks, computerised robots (for welding, etc.) and a greater concern for the physical work environment have reduced the amount of heavy lifting and have improved ergonomic conditions. However, despite considerable ergonomic improvements in work conditions in the industrialised countries, MSD have remained a major health problem and to some extent have even increased (EU Working Conditions Survey, 2006; European Agency for Safety and Health at Work, 2010). Neck and shoulder problems are reported frequently among workers in Europe and North America, and this is also an increasing problem in economically developed countries such as Japan and South Korea. Pain symptoms are often also reported in light physical work, for example in computerised jobs, in assembly work in the electronic industry and among workers at call centres answering telephone calls. In these jobs, employees are probably using only 1–2% of their maximal capacity or even less, and therefore it is unlikely that the high prevalence of MSD — and neck and shoulder pain in particular — can be explained by excessive muscle load. Physical strength as such is not linked to the risk of muscle pain symptoms in these types of jobs, and in modern workstations the ergonomic conditions are usually quite good.

MSD and stress

In a number of studies it has been found that psychosocial conditions at work, such as mental stress, are related to MSD (Linton, 2002; Johansson *et al.*, 2003). In cross-sectional studies investigating symptoms as well as work conditions, it is likely that a 'negative response bias' may influence the results. For example, workers suffering from muscle pain are probably more likely to report stressful work conditions compared with workers without symptoms. The fact that workers suffering from musculoskeletal symptoms also report more negative work conditions means that they suffer from a 'double burden': both pain and low job satisfaction. However, a number of longitudinal studies (Bigos *et al.*, 1991; Leino & Magni, 1993) have also been performed, and have confirmed that psychosocial factors such as work stress and lack of job satisfaction are related to increased muscular pain 5–10 years later. Recently, Canivet *et al.* (2008) found that sleeping problems were related to more musculoskeletal problems one year later in initially healthy working women and men. Job strain was also independently and significantly predictive of musculoskeletal pain in women, but synergistic effects between sleeping problems and job strain were small. A reasonable explanation for the findings by Canivet *et al.* is that sleeping problems disturb anabolic processes during sleep, prevent muscle relaxation and healing, and activate the part of the brain involved in pain modulation. As pain is also likely to induce sleep problems, this may start a vicious circle.

These findings indicate that other, non-biomechanical factors may be of importance for the development of muscular pain. This is supported by a series of recent studies showing that psychosocial factors at work, such as stress, lack of job satisfaction, dysfunctional work organisation, injustice and so on, have been linked to neck, shoulder and back pain problems. Mehlum *et al.* (2008) investigated occupational factors assumed to be relevant for socio-economic inequalities in musculoskeletal pain, finding that physical demands explained a large part of occupational class inequalities in back pain, but that lack of job autonomy was more important for inequalities in neck–shoulder pain and arm pain. This is consistent with general findings on the relationship between work-related stress and MSD, showing that back pain is more strongly related to physical work conditions and neck and shoulder pain to mental stress at work.

The trapezius muscle, which covers the neck, the shoulders and the upper part of the back, is of particular interest as it represents the area where most people contract pain disorders. The influence of mental stress on stress hormones, blood pressure, heart rate and other biomarkers of stress is well known, whereas information about the influence of mental stress on muscle activity was limited until a couple of decades ago. In several laboratory experiments it has now been shown that mental stress, without any physical activity, has a significant effect on activity in the trapezius muscle. Active muscle fibres generate electrical activity, which can be recorded with suitable electrodes. The trapezius muscle is located just under the skin, and electrical signals from this muscle can easily be recorded by surface electrodes attached to the skin. By exposing an individual to mental stress, for example mental arithmetic and other cognitive tasks, it has been demonstrated that the electrical activity from the trapezius muscle, measured by electromyography (EMG), increases in the same way as in response to physical demands (Lundberg *et al.*,1994, 2002; Wærsted, 1997; Krantz *et al.*, 2004). The magnitude of the stress-induced response is comparable to what has been seen in office work, for example sitting at a computer, where a lot of people develop neck and shoulder pain (Fig. 6.4).

Devereux *et al.* (2004) performed a prospective study of 3139 workers for 15 months and found that high perceived job stress mediated a relation between exposure to high physical and psychosocial work conditions and self-reported MSD. It was concluded that interventions aimed at reducing musculoskeletal complaints need to take both physical and psychosocial work risk factors into consideration. Miranda *et al.* (2008) followed 2256 blue- and white-collar workers free of low-back pain for 12 months and found that workers of different ages were affected by different factors. Physical workload (heavy lifting, awkward postures, whole-body vibration) predicted low-back pain in workers under 50 years of age, whereas unhealthy behaviours (smoking, overweight, lack of physical exercise) predicted low-back pain in workers 50 years and older. Mental stress, dissatisfaction and sleep problems significantly predicted low-back pain in the age group 40–49 years. Laursen *et al.* (2002) measured muscular activity (EMG) from the forearm and neck muscles during computer mouse work with two levels of mental demands and found that mental demands increased muscular activity in all recorded muscles. Buckle and Devereux (2002) reviewed the epidemiological evidence for the work-relatedness of neck and upper limb MSD and concluded that there is a relationship between the performance of work and such disorders and that interventions for the reduction of these disorders should involve the work organisation as well as the individual worker. They also concluded that current knowledge is sufficient for the design of preventive strategies at the societal, organisational and

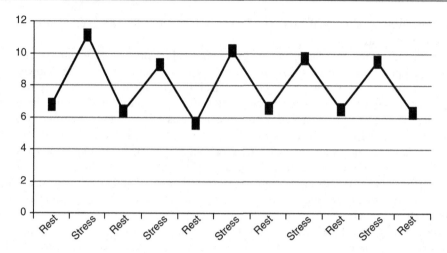

Fig. 6.4 Muscle activity (EMG) in response to repeated mental stress (% of reference level). Reprinted from Lundberg *et al.* (2002) with permission.

individual level. Vingård *et al.* (2000) compared 695 persons seeking care for back pain with 1423 matched referents and found that the combination of high physical and high psychosocial stress at work increased the risk for back pain substantially. Hoogendoorn *et al.* (2001) examined 861 workers from 34 companies in The Netherlands during a 3-year follow-up period and concluded that low social support at work was a risk factor for low-back pain. Similarly, Elfering, Semmer, Schade *et al.* (2002) found that low supervisor support increased the risk of low back pain in 46 initially healthy individuals followed up over 5 years, but that high support from a closest colleague had a detrimental effect. Elfering, Gregner *et al.* (2002) investigated the role of mental work stressors on the development of back pain in 114 nurses during a one-year period. Lack of time control (external locus of control) at the beginning of the study predicted low-back pain one year later. In a subsample of nurses, urinary catecholamines were measured and adrenaline as well as noradrenaline levels were found to be higher in participants with more frequent episodes of back pain. By examining predictors of lumbar disc degeneration in healthy individuals followed up for 5 years, it was found that physical and psychological job characteristics were more important than the clinical magnetic resonance imaging (MRI) investigations in predicting the need for medical consultation and work incapacity (Boos *et al.*, 2000) and that lack of sports activities and working on the night shift were significant risk factors for the development of disc generation (Elfering, Semmer, Birkhofer *et al.*, 2002). Wergeland *et al.* (2003) found that the shortening of regular workdays from 7 hours or more to 6 hours significantly reduced the prevalence of neck–shoulder pain in workers with physically demanding care work.

Women usually report more symptoms than men, and this gender difference cannot be explained only by differences in muscular strength. The gender differences are most pronounced among white-collar workers, who are usually exposed to very low physical demands. Gender differences also exist in jobs where women and men are performing the same tasks. Nordander *et al.* (1999) compared 116 male and 206 female workers employed in fish processing plants, who were required to perform the same task and who had a high risk of neck and upper limb disorders. It was found that women workers in the fish industry had a higher prevalence of complaints of the neck and shoulder than their male co-workers. The reason for these gender differences is not clear, but even in the same job men and women may be exposed differently. For example, Nordander *et al.* (2008) found that women reported more repetitiveness, more constrained neck postures and a more stressful work environment than did men. Another possibility is that women are more vulnerable, not only because of their lower muscular strength, which is likely to be of importance in jobs involving more heavy work, e.g. in many caring jobs, but also because of gender differences in muscle fibre composition or stress sensitivity. In a small experimental study (Krantz *et al.*, 2002), it was found that the relationship between stress-induced EMG activity in the trapezius and cardiovascular stress responses was much stronger in women than in men, which indicates that women's muscular responses are more strongly related to mental stress than are men's. In a study by Silverstein *et al.* (2009) of 733 individuals in 12 healthcare and manufacturing workplaces, gender differences in response to physical work exposures were considered to reflect gender segregation in work conditions and physical capacity (pinch and lifting). Marras *et al.* (2000) found that psychosocial stress increased lumbar spine load more in women than in men and that certain personality traits were associated with increased spine loading.

The mechanisms causing muscular pain in heavy physical work are quite well known. Less is known about the mechanisms linking low muscular activity to pain symptoms. In office work, tasks performed at the computer, assembly work in the electronic industry, and work at call centres, neck and shoulder pain is a common problem, despite the fact that the workers use only a fraction of their maximal muscular capacity. This indicates that there is no lower limit of muscular activity that is 'safe'. Even low levels of muscular activity for long periods of time may cause pain problems. In order to explain these relationships, a number of models have been developed.

Explanatory models

According to Schleifer and Ley (1994), mental stress induces hyperventilation, which changes the blood chemistry. Hyperventilation (i.e. breathing more than necessary for metabolic reasons) reduces carbon dioxide levels, among other things, and the blood becomes more alkaline which induces muscle tension and a greater sensitivity to stress hormones. Another suggestion by Knardahl (2002) is based on the interaction between blood vessels and nerves during stress-induced muscle tension. Muscle tension means stretching of blood vessels, which increases the secretion of pain-inducing substances such as prosta-glandins. This process is similar to what is supposed to happen during a migraine attack.

Johansson and his colleagues (2003) have proposed a theory based on the sensory organs embedded in the muscles, the 'muscle spindles'. These are coordinating movements allocating muscle activity in relation to the demands. The density of muscle spindles is particularly high in the trapezius muscle, an area where most people develop pain syndromes. In response to mental stress, static load and repetitive physical activity, sympathetic modulation of muscle spindles has been found to be dysfunctional. The muscle spindles send signals to the muscles to increase the force, and the stiff muscles send signals back that more strength is necessary, which may start a vicious circle eventually leading to chronic pain. In stiff muscles blood flow is reduced and metabolites and pain-inducing substances may accumulate, which induces additional pain and inflammatory activity.

Another model is based on the smallest functional units of the muscle, the 'motor units'. A motor unit consists of a number of muscle fibres, which are all activated by one nerve signal. Each muscle consists of a number of motor units, and the more force that is necessary the more motor units are activated. In the trapezius muscle it has been demonstrated that the recruitment of motor units occurs in a specific order (Henneman *et al.*, 1965). At low levels of force, small motor units with low thresholds are active first. When force increases, larger units with higher thresholds are recruited in an orderly fashion. When force decreases, the motor units are derecruited in the opposite order. This means that motor units recruited first are active until the muscle is completely relaxed. This is an important component of the 'Cinderella Hypothesis' (Hägg, 1991). Cinderella in the fairy tale was the person who had to get up first in the morning to work and the last one to go to bed. According to the hypothesis the small, low-threshold motor units are active as long as the muscle is at all activated. This means that during long-term exposure to low levels of force, these motor units and the muscle fibres belonging to them will be continuously active, which may cause metabolic disturbances, damaged muscle fibres ('red ragged fibres'), accumulation of metabolites and other pain-inducing substances and eventually cause chronic pain. If damaged muscle fibres are continuously active, there is no time for healing processes, which is an additional problem. Another factor of importance is that in jobs with low levels of force, such as work at the computer or at call centres, there are usually no signs of fatigue, which means that the individual can continue to work for hours and days without knowing that certain small motor units are exhausted. Continuous low muscle activity may also cause pain as a result of active muscle fibres chafing passive muscle fibres.

These theories differ to some extent and overlap in some cases. There is empirical support for all of them, and additional explanatory models have been proposed. However, the models are complementary rather than contradictory, and it seems likely that there are different mechanisms that explain the development of muscle pain in different individuals and in different situations. A common feature of the models, however, is that mental stress has an important role and contributes to the pathogenic processes. In the same vein, it has been demonstrated that mental stress may activate the same motor units as physical activity (Lundberg *et al.*, 2002). This means that, if the worker is unable to relax mentally, mental stress may keep the same group of muscle fibres as active as physical demands, preventing muscle rest not only during work but also during breaks and outside work. As mental stress usually is more long-lasting and more difficult to get rid of, stressful work is likely to be an important problem in the development of MSD in jobs with low physical demands but high psychosocial stress, a type of employment that is increasing in all parts of the world (Fig. 6.5).

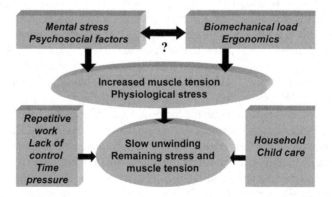

Fig. 6.5 A model for musculoskeletal disorders. Based on Melin & Lundberg (1997) with permission.

ULCERS

For a long time peptic ulcers were considered to be caused by stress and an unhealthy diet, and patients were treated with surgery, a strict diet and stress-monitoring programmes. The role of stress for this disease was questioned after two Australian researchers, Warren and Marshall demonstrated in 1983 that it is caused by a bacterium, *Helicobacter pylori*, and can be treated by antibiotics. Nevertheless, Sapolsky (1998) chose ulcers as an example of a stress-related disorder that adversely affects humans but seldom animals. An important point raised by Sapolsky is that *Helicobacter* cannot be the only explanation for this disorder as more than 50% of the world's population harbour this bacterium in their gastrointestinal tract but only about 20% of those infected show symptoms. This means that other factors are involved. According to Sapolsky, stress is such a factor. Under stressful conditions gastrointestinal activity is reduced. Saliva production is reduced, and the stomach and the intestines are less active and not prepared for food intake. In order not to waste 'unnecessary' energy when the stress systems are activated, the mucosa of the inner surface of the stomach wall becomes thinner and more vulnerable to damage by the hydrochloric acid in the stomach. A weaker mucous layer opens the possibility for *Helicobacter pylori* to more easily penetrate the lining of the stomach, to invade the stomach wall and cause ulcers. According to Sapolsky, 30–65% of peptic ulcers are estimated to be associated with psychosocial factors such as stress. Generally, studies indicate that ulcers are formed during recovery after a stressful period.

HIV, AIDS AND CANCER

In patients infected with human immunodeficiency virus (HIV), there is a successive decline in the functioning of the immune system, eventually resulting in its complete breakdown and the acquired immunodeficiency syndrome (AIDS). Individual differences in the progress of this disease have contributed to an interest in the role of depression and stress for the disease course of HIV patients. Moskowitz (2003) found that positive affect predicted lower risk of AIDS mortality after 12–24 months in 407 men who were HIV-positive at study baseline. Leserman (2008) has summarised a large body of evidence on the effects of depression and stress on immune- and disease-related parameters in HIV patients, finding substantial support for a relation between chronic depression and stressful events, HIV disease progression and a protective role for social support. Less is known about the possible biological mechanisms involved, but Antoni *et al.* (2002) investigated the effects of a 10-week stress management intervention programme in 25 HIV-infected men and found that men receiving stress management had improved their immunological functioning compared with what happened in patients in the control condition without intervention. The positive effects of stress management have been demonstrated in addition to the effects of antiretroviral medication, which also inhibits the progression of HIV. Similar findings were reported by Carrico *et al.* (2005), who examined the effects of a cognitive behavioural stress management intervention on HIV-infected gay men. They found that the intervention contributed to better psychosocial status and immunological control of latent Epstein-Barr virus, which may accelerate HIV disease progression.

The immune system, and the natural killer (NK) cells in particular, are assumed to play an important function in attacking and killing cancer cells. Epidemiological studies indicate that stress, chronic depression and lack of social support might serve as risk factors for cancer development and progression, but there is little rigorous evidence of stress causing cancer (Sapolsky, 1998). Stress hormones can modulate the activity of the tumour and promote tumour-cell growth, and can also activate viruses, altering the immune function to create a more permissive environment for tumour growth. Reviews of recent cellular and molecular studies have identified biological processes that could potentially mediate such effects (Antoni *et al.*, 2006). A possible mechanism supported by animal theories is that chronic stress promotes formation of new blood vessels that feed tumours, and thus stimulates growth and the more rapid spread of tumours (Thaker *et al.*, 2006). In addition, psychological stress has been found to reduce the efficacy of chemotherapy in breast cancer patients (Su *et al.*, 2005).

WHEN SHOULD I BE WORRIED?

Various symptoms, such as temporary muscle pain, palpitation, distress, anxiety, sleep problems, headaches and stomachache, occur frequently in most people without being indications of serious illness or disease. These symptoms usually disappear after some time regardless of treatment. Thus, in most cases minor symptoms are natural and usually harmless. However, when a great number of symptoms start to appear within a relatively short period of time, and this happens after a period of long-lasting or intense stress exposure, these symptoms should serve as important warning signals. If no actions are taken to treat them and to prevent exposure to additional stress, more severe stress-related conditions could develop, such as burnout syndrome, PTSD, chronic fatigue, depression and fibromyalgia. Counteractive measures should include opportunities for rest, recuperation, regular, moderate and pleasant physical activity, and sleep, but this is usually not possible without major changes to the individual's occupational and life situation. More discussion on interventions to prevent stress-related disorders and promote occupational health will be presented in Chapter 9.

Typical symptoms

Typical symptoms that frequently occur in association with chronic stress are:

- Impaired performance.
- Lack of motivation ('What used to be fun isn't fun any more').
- Problems concentrating and staying focused.
- Memory problems.
- Diffuse pain in the body.
- Sleep problems (difficulty going to sleep, fragmented sleep, early wake-up or excessive sleep without feeling recuperated).
- Frequent or long-lasting infections.
- Chest pain.
- Palpitations.
- Oversensitivity.
- Dizziness.

These symptoms could indicate that the regulation of important bodily systems is disturbed. In some cases, long-term exposure to stress results in serious disorders that appear very suddenly and may resemble a heart attack. Symptoms such chest pain, very high blood pressure, partial paralysis (e.g. not being able to move arms or legs), difficulties breathing and speaking, dizziness and the feeling of dying are common. When taken to hospital, the first thing that doctors do is exclude serious CVD (infarction, stroke).

HOW CAN ANY TREATMENT BE EFFICIENT?

As minor symptoms come and go, people may associate their improved health with their own actions taken during illness, even if the association occurred by chance. Different forms of self-treatment appear (taking herbal medicine, wearing warm clothing, having a hot bath, staying in bed, drinking green tea, etc.). This phenomenon also opens the possibility for non-evidence-based (alternative) treatments, which are still scientifically in doubt. People usually seek help when their symptoms are most severe. Since symptoms vary in intensity over time, a decline in severity can be expected after a peak, and by introduction of any kind of treatment at that point (efficient or not), a positive outcome is likely to follow which 'confirms' the efficacy of the treatment. Additional positive placebo effects from alternative treatments seem to be obtained if the method is claimed to be based on traditional oriental medicine with a thousand-year-old history and a holistic approach (We treat the person, not the symptom), are said to be able to treat almost any disorder (from distress and muscle pain to heart disease and cancer), involve physical contact with the patient, and are expensive (inexpensive treatment is usually perceived as less effective). This phenomenon creates opportunities to do profitable business with almost any kind of non-tested pill or treatment.

7 Stress Hormones at Work

Stress hormones constitute an 'objective' measure of stress at work, and are therefore often used as biomarkers of occupational stress. These measures are not biased by potentially negative or positive attitudes towards the work situation by the employer or trade union, which may be the case for some self-reported stress measures. Self-reports may also be influenced by unconscious factors. For example, it is likely that workers who are suffering from various symptoms that they believe are work-related would rate their work situation more negatively compared with workers without symptoms. Stress hormones also constitute an important link between psychosocial stress and various health problems as described in Chapter 6.

As stress hormones are secreted into the blood stream, the levels can be measured by sampling and analysing blood. This is a direct measure of the momentary circulating levels of stress hormones in the body. However, blood sampling is not always possible or convenient, especially when studying stress in natural settings such as in the workplace. Blood sampling requires trained medical personnel, and the punctuation of a blood vessel to sample blood can be a stressor in itself and can cause an increase in stress hormone secretion. This means that the method of investigation contributes to elevated stress hormone levels and the results may reflect the stress of the investigation rather than normal stress levels at work. Another problem with measurements in blood is that stress hormone levels in blood fluctuate rapidly and may differ between different sampling sites and between venous and arterial blood. Therefore, in order to obtain a reliable measure reflecting the normal stress hormone level in blood on a work day, repeated or continuous sampling is necessary. This can be done by means of a catheter. If this catheter is inserted before measurements start, the individual habituates and the stress from the insertion of the catheter diminishes over time. In a laboratory situation this is an adequate method, but it is seldom possible to perform normal work with a needle in the arm and thus measuring stress hormones in blood could give a very inaccurate picture of the influence of a normal work situation on stress level.

Before 1960, stress hormones could only be reliably measured in blood (or plasma), but the demonstration that a relatively constant proportion of the stress hormones in blood is also excreted into urine made it possible to estimate circulating stress hormone levels in blood from urine samples (von Euler & Lishajko, 1961; Frankenhaeuser, 1971). Collecting urine samples is not usually stressful or harmful, and does not interfere very much with the

The Science of Occupational Health: Stress, Psychobiology and the New World of Work, first edition
By Ulf Lundberg and Cary L. Cooper. Published 2011 by Blackwell Publishing Ltd
© 2011 Ulf Lundberg and Cary L. Cooper

individual's normal environment and conditions. Another advantage when studying work stress is that urine samples naturally produce an integrated mean measure of circulating stress hormones for the period under which the urine sample was produced. For example, if the worker is emptying the bladder upon arrival at work at 9 am in the morning and then a urine sample is collected at 12 noon, the amount of stress hormones reveals the average stress level during this period. The advantage of using urinary measures for the study of work stress resulted in a rapid expansion of research on stress hormone levels at work from the beginning of the 1960s (review by Lundberg, 1984).

The concentration of stress hormones in urine depends on the amount of fluid in the bladder. Drinking a lot of water or other liquids dilutes the sample. Therefore, in order to estimate the total amount of stress hormone secretion for a particular period of time, the total volume of urine produced during the time between testing has to be measured. The hormone assay is usually performed on a small subsample of urine, and the total amount of hormones excreted is estimated by multiplying the amount in the subsample by the total urine volume. If stress hormones in urine samples produced during different time periods are compared, the time between emptying of the bladder also has to be considered. Therefore, a normal procedure to estimate stress hormones in urine involves measurements of the total urine volume produced, and of the number of minutes that had passed since the previous emptying of the bladder. The concentration of stress hormones assessed from the subsample is then multiplied by the total volume of urine and divided by the number of minutes. This measure is usually expressed in number of picomoles per minute, which can be compared between individuals and between conditions. In order to protect the stress hormones from decay, the urine sample has to be frozen until analysed and for adrenaline and noradrenaline also acidified to a pH level of about 3.0. In order to estimate the effects of the work situation as such on stress hormone levels, a number of confounders have to be taken into consideration and controlled for. The most important are diurnal and seasonal variations, medication, cigarette smoking and alcohol intake.

The stress hormone cortisol, but so far neither adrenaline nor noradrenaline, can be measured in blood and urine and also in saliva. Measurements in saliva have the same advantages as urine samples in that they do not influence the natural work situation very much and do not induce pain or distress, which could give misleading results. Furthermore, saliva samples can be obtained more frequently than urine samples, they reflect free (active) cortisol and are independent of saliva flow. Another practical advantage is that saliva samples can be stored in room temperature for up to three weeks without deterioration (Garde & Hansen, 2005). This makes it possible to perform studies in which the participants are instructed to collect and store saliva themselves for several days. Saliva samples are often obtained using plastic containers (e.g. Salivette tubes) with a cotton swab, which the participants are instructed to put in their mouth for a couple of minutes until it is soaked with saliva. The cotton swab is then put back into the container and the saliva samples can be returned to the experimenters even by regular mail. It is also possible to spit directly into the plastic container. Other means of saliva sampling can also be used, for example paper strips. In order to obtain reliable results it is of utmost importance that the participants comply with the instructions. Even minor deviations in terms of when the sample is taken, particularly in the morning when cortisol levels vary rapidly, can cause great differences and seriously bias the results.

In order to study stress at work, comparisons are usually made between stress hormone levels at work and corresponding measures at the same time of day on a non-work day, thus controlling for diurnal variation in hormone secretion and at the same time controlling for individual differences in normal hormonal levels. Adrenaline and noradrenaline levels follow a sinusoidal pattern, with low levels during night sleep and a peak in the middle of the day. Noradrenaline levels depend very much on physical activity, whereas adrenaline circadian rhythm is relatively stable even during sleep deprivation. Cortisol levels peak early in the morning, in saliva about 30 min after awakening, and then decline during the day and the evening, with moderate peaks after lunch and dinner. Cortisol levels are low during night sleep but start to increase in the morning before waking up. Deviations from this normal pattern can be caused by acute or chronic stress (high workload, intense emotions), altered sleep patterns (shift and night work, east–west flights and jet lag) and various forms of medication. Stress hormones have also been found to vary in relation to season. Hansen *et al.* (2001) compared urinary adrenaline, noradrenaline and cortisol levels over a year in 11 healthy females and found that concentrations of urinary adrenaline were higher during June and July, and urinary cortisol during December and January, compared with the rest of the year. Urinary excretion of norepinephrine was higher during working hours and lower during the evening from August to May, compared with June and July. Possible explanations for these variations are the length of day (daylight) and variations in physical activity. Temperature, psychosocial stress and menstrual cycle could not explain this seasonal variation in stress hormones (Hansen, Garde, Skovgaard & Christensen, 2001). Persson *et al.* (2008) investigated seasonal variation in human salivary cortisol concentration in 24 individuals (men and women) and found the highest concentrations in February, March and April, and the lowest in July and August. Differences in study design may contribute to some variation in results, but studies are generally consistent in finding that cortisol levels are higher during winter than in the summer.

Inter-individual variation in urinary catecholamines and salivary cortisol is quite large but intra-individual levels are relatively stable over time (Lundberg & Forsman, 1980; Hansen, Garde, Christensen *et al.*, 2001). The normal inter-individual range of variation in, for example, urinary adrenaline levels is about 1:10 between the lowest and the highest in a random sample of individuals. Salivary cortisol levels vary even more between individuals. This means that direct comparisons between groups of individuals working under different conditions have to be based on a large sample of individuals to reach an adequate statistical power. By making intra-individual comparisons, that is, by comparing the same group of workers at their jobs and on a non-work day, the influence of a particular work situation in one organisation on stress levels can be compared with corresponding measures in another type of organisation, using a relatively small sample of employees. With this approach a great number of successful studies have been performed on groups of 20–30 employees. For example, Frankenhaeuser *et al.* (1989) compared 30 male and 30 female white-collar workers on and off the job and found, among other things, that both men and women increased their adrenaline levels significantly at work but that women's stress levels tended also to remain elevated after work. Similar findings have been reported by Lundberg and Frankenhaeuser (1999) with 30 male and 30 female managers.

In this way, it is possible to compare how different working conditions are associated with different psychological and biological stress responses. A typical finding among white-collar workers is that adrenaline levels increase about 50–100% at work compared with non-work levels, whereas noradrenaline and cortisol increase very little or not at all in white-collar workers during stable normal work conditions (Lundberg & Frankenhaeuser, 1999; Pollard, 1995). Among blue-collar workers, adrenaline levels may increase even more and, at the same time, noradrenaline levels are elevated (e.g. Lundberg *et al.*, 1989; Melin *et al.*, 1999; Lundberg & Johansson, 2000). Individual differences in responses to work-related stress are great, even in the same work environment, which may reflect individual differences in resources to cope with stress and/or the fact that certain work conditions are perceived as more stressful by some individuals than by others. Nevertheless, work conditions defined as 'high strain' jobs according to the Demand–Control model or stressful in terms of Effort–Reward Imbalance, usually induce higher stress levels in most individuals compared with work conditions defined as less stressful according to these theories.

Cortisol levels increase very little or not at all during normal routine office work. However, unexpected and emotional events, such as reorganisations, new management, conflicts and threats of closing down and/or of unemployment, may evoke increased cortisol secretion. Cortisol levels also increase when the individual expects a heavy workload, long working hours and emotional stress. Hansen *et al.* (2006) found significantly higher salivary cortisol levels in construction workers compared with a reference group of white-collar workers, and the increase in cortisol had already started on waking before going to work. This shows that anticipation of a heavy workload induces physiological activity, which prepares the body for coping with the expected demands during the working day. Steptoe *et al.* (2000) found a significant elevation in salivary cortisol early in the working day in male and female teachers ($n = 105$), which was greater in teachers with high job strain according to the Demand–Control model.

Elevated cortisol levels in the morning have also been found after insufficient sleep during the night (Ekstedt *et al.*, 2004), and among employees who do not feel recovered after a night's sleep (Gustafsson *et al.*, 2008). This is likely to be a normal healthy response which helps the individual to mobilise energy to cope with expected daily hassles or compensate for lack of restitution during the night, and is not, in the short term, associated with any particular health risks. Long-term activation of these systems, on the other hand, may contribute to a great number of stress-related health problems as described in Chapter 6.

In jobs characterised by repetitive work tasks, stress responses seem to remain elevated even after work (Melin *et al.*, 1999; Lundberg & Johansson, 2000), which means that workers are also exposed to high stress hormone levels, high heart rate, high blood pressure, elevated blood lipids, etc. during breaks at work and in the evening after work. The reason for this after-effect is not quite clear, but could be explained by the more negative stress induced by repetitive work tasks and lack of influence and control, which makes it difficult to relax after work in the evening at home. Also, workers in repetitive jobs usually have a lower income and less education compared with white-collar workers, which could be interpreted as a chronic stressor and associated with generally elevated adrenaline and cortisol levels (Cohen *et al.*, 2006). It could also be that repetitive work tasks induce more long-lasting stress compared with more flexible and variable work tasks (Frankenhaeuser, 1986). The association between stress levels on and off work is usually stronger in women than in men. Biological stress responses in male workers (stress hormones, blood pressure) are usually significantly related to their perceived stress at work, whereas women's workload and biological responses at work are also correlated with their stress levels after work and during the weekend (Lundberg, 1996). More on gender differences in work, stress and health is presented in Chapter 10.

8 Socioeconomic Status and Health

An association between low socioeconomic status (SES) and poor health exists in all parts of the world (Black *et al.*, 1980; Kawachi & Kennedy, 2002; Östlin, 2004; Marmot, 2008). SES is often defined in terms of education, occupational position and income, but, as shown by Geyer *et al.* (2006), correlations between these measures are low or moderate and thus each measure contains specific information related to health outcomes. In poor countries, physical conditions such as lack of medical care, inadequate nutrition, polluted water, bad housing and poor sanitary conditions are important explanations for ill health, but in affluent societies other factors linked to SES, such as relative deprivation, lifestyles and behaviours (smoking, alcohol, unhealthy dietary habits, lack of exercise, violence, etc.), work conditions and access to social networks, may contribute to health irregularities (Lundberg & Fritzell, 1994; Adler *et al.*, 1999; Marmot, 2004). Access to health care could be of importance for SES differences in health, but these differences exist also in countries with free or almost free access to health care, and only a small part of the SES–health relationship can be explained by lifestyle factors. Well known demonstrations of a systematic social gradient in health come from the Whitehall studies led by Professor Sir Michael Marmot (Marmot *et al.*, 1978). The Whitehall studies are long-term investigations of the influences on health of circumstances at work, at home and in the wider community. The first Whitehall study of 18 000 British male civil servants between the ages of 20 and 64 was set up in 1967, and showed that men in the lowest employment grades were much more likely to die prematurely than men in the highest grades. The Whitehall II study, with more than 10 000 participants (both women and men), was set up in 1985 to determine the conditions that underlie this social gradient in death and disease. The results from these studies, consistently showing that people in lower social positions have worse health and shorter life expectancy than those who are more favoured, have been published widely in scientific journals and books. These results have also become part of general policy discussions and have contributed to strategies to improve health in several European countries (Whitehead *et al.*, 1999; Östlin & Diderichsen, 2001; Mackenbach *et al.*, 2003). On the basis of general statistics from England and Wales during the period 1999–2003, Romeri *et al.* (2006) calculated relative deprivation scores (20 categories) based on material conditions (car ownership), occupational status (unemployed, low job status) and social conditions (overcrowding). Deprivation scores were significantly related to age-standardised all-cause mortality in males and females. Mortality in the most

The Science of Occupational Health: Stress, Psychobiology and the New World of Work, first edition
By Ulf Lundberg and Cary L. Cooper. Published 2011 by Blackwell Publishing Ltd
© 2011 Ulf Lundberg and Cary L. Cooper

deprived group was more than 2.5 times higher than that in the least deprived. The leading causes of death were CVD (CHD, stroke) and cancer. In countries such as Sweden, where SES differences are considered to be relatively small, a strong social gradient in health exists (Statistics Sweden, 2008).

It is generally concluded that psychosocial factors have increasing importance for health differences in different social groups, and subjective SES is as important as objective SES. This means that the individual's perceived social, occupational and economic status in society has a direct influence on his or her mental and physical health. It has been proposed that the same low SES predicts poorer health in countries and communities with a greater income inequality, compared with societies with a more narrow range of income (Wilkinson, 2000; Wilkinson & Pickett, 2009). However, the strong negative correlation found between income inequality and life expectancy in nine Western industrialised countries by Wilkinson in 1992, which was replicated in studies of differences in mortality between states in the USA, has been questioned and considered as an artefact of the selection of countries and states (Mackenbach, 2002). This critical view is supported by a Japanese study (Shibuya *et al.*, 2002), based on nationally representative samples from each prefecture, which showed that individual income was more strongly related to self-rated health than income inequality. Similarly, Sturm and Gresenz (2002) found an association between health and education or family income in 60 metropolitan areas in the USA, but no evidence for a relationship between income inequality and physical and mental disorders. Muller (2002) concluded, in a study of all USA states including Washington DC, that lack of high-school education accounts for the income inequality effect and is a strong predictor of mortality in the USA. However, more recently Wilkinson and Pickett (2009) presented statistics showing that economic inequality within countries still seems to be a greater health problem than mean differences in economy between countries. On almost every index of quality of life, there is a gradient showing a strong relation between a country's level of economic inequality and its social outcomes. Wilkinson and Pickett (2009) emphasise the importance of hierarchy and status, and contend that inequality causes shorter, unhealthier and unhappier lives, which may explain why people in unequal societies, such as UK and USA (countries that usually end up on the negative side), have a shorter lifespan compared with more egalitarian countries such as Japan and Sweden (countries that usually end up on the positive side). However, as indicated above, other differences between these countries can also be of importance, such as access to affordable health care, social welfare systems, housing conditions, criminality and the proportion of the population living in poverty. Thus, the relationship between SES and health is complex and multifactorial (Marmot, 2008), and the role of relative versus absolute deprivation is not clear. Nevertheless, many of the factors involved are stress related.

Working conditions are likely to have a particularly important role for health equity (Marmot & Wilkinson, 2006). This is dramatically illustrated by data from the Whitehall I study in the UK (Fig. 8.1; Marmot & Shipley, 1996), showing that mortality among male civil servants aged 40–64 years with manual work roles is four times higher compared with upper managers and administrators, despite the fact that civil servants constitute a relatively homogeneous group in which employees tend to have a secure job and the same access to health care. It is of particular interest that, in the Whitehall study, the risk of dying followed a gradient on which office workers had about three times higher the risk of dying and middle managers about two times higher compared with senior managers and administrators. Work can be 'health promoting' by providing financial security, social status, personal development, social relationships and self-esteem. However, work conditions can also cause health problems. Negative work conditions, such as lack of an interesting job, exposure to adverse

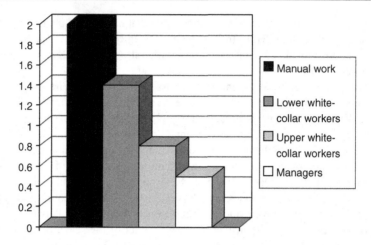

Fig. 8.1 Mortality (relative risk) and occupational status among British Civil Servants (40–64 years); 25-year follow-up of the Whitehall Study. Based on Marmot & Shipley (1996) with permission.

working conditions, health hazards and low pay, are factors that often characterise low-status jobs, usually performed by workers with low education levels. This means that poor education and low-status jobs interact with a cluster of factors known to cause health problems. In addition to physical hazards, low-status jobs often involve high job demands, low control and effort–reward imbalance (Stansfeld & Candy, 2006), which, according to the most established occupational stress theories, is strongly linked to mental and physical health problems. Furthermore, low social and economic status seems to constitute a risk factor of its own.

Matthews *et al.* (2000) investigated 50 men and 50 women, pair-wise matched for occupational status, and found that individuals in low-prestige occupations experienced more interpersonal conflict, greater arousal and higher heart rate. On the basis of data from 125 men and 96 women from the Whitehall II Study, Steptoe *et al.* (2003a) found that low job control was related to greater fibrinogen stress responses in men but not in women. As high fibrinogen level is a risk factor for CVD, this could be one mechanism explaining the relation between low occupational status and CVD risk. The lack of association in women was assumed to be due to hormone replacement therapy. Gallo *et al.* (2004) measured occupational status and ambulatory systolic blood pressure and heart rate in 180 women for two days. They found that occupational status predicted cardiovascular activity after controlling for a number of possible confounders. It was concluded that the higher cardiovascular risk associated with lower status occupations and stressful jobs could be due to elevated cardiovascular activity. Similarly, Steptoe *et al.* (2003b) found higher morning systolic blood pressure in lower grade participants in the Whitehall II Study. As demonstrated by Wamala (1999), there is a strong social gradient in CHD in women, stronger than for men, showing that women with unskilled or semiskilled occupations had a fourfold increased risk of developing CHD compared with women executives and professionals.

In a review by Sapolsky (2005) summarising findings on the physiological mediators of the social position–health relationship in different species, the author concludes that stress-induced health problems related to social position depend on the stability of the social hierarchy. In relatively stable social hierarchies such as in humans, rats and mice, where subordinates are exposed to social stressors and low availability of social support, low social rank gives rise to a particular psychophysiological profile with high levels of stress hormones and low levels of anabolic sex hormones. An association based on a reverse causal order is unlikely, as studies show that psychophysiological profiles of single animals do not predict their subsequent ranks in social groups (Sapolsky, 2005). In social groups where dominance has to be repeatedly and physically defended (e.g. among male chimpanzees), high social status is associated with elevated physiological arousal and increased disease risk, which is in line with the health risks associated with allostatic load in response to unremitting stress (McEwen & Lasley, 2002).

In humans, measurements of social position or rank are more complex than in animals. For example, humans may belong to several hierarchies. An individual in a low-status job, or with a low level of education, may be a top player in a football team or a great singer and receive a lot of prestige in those other roles. In addition, parental SES seems to influence children's health status (Evans, 2004; Goodman et al., 2005), and also has an effect when they become adults (Vågerö & Leon, 1994). Thus, the psychophysiological mechanisms linking SES to health in humans can be expected to be multifactorial. Measures of social standing, income, education and rank in social hierarchies may also differ. Nevertheless, the SES–health associations are very robust in humans (Kawachi & Kennedy, 2002).

Low SES can be considered as a moderate but chronically stressful condition that influences the major bodily stress systems (Cohen et al., 2006). Differences in allostatic load may reflect differences in stress exposure, and constitute a link between SES and health differences (Szanton et al., 2005). Activity in the sympathetic adrenal medullary system (secretion of adrenaline and noradrenaline) and the HPA axis (secretion of cortisol) is thus likely to play a key role (Henry & Stephens, 1977). The cortisol awakening response, and the difference between morning and evening values, seem to be of particular importance (Gunnar & Vazquez, 2001; Clow et al., 2004). In monkeys and rodents, high social status is usually associated with high levels of sex hormones (testosterone in males) and low levels of cortisol/corticosterone, whereas low-status animals display an opposite pattern (Sapolsky, 1998). In agreement with animal research (Henry, 1992), the HPA axis has been suggested to reflect social status in humans also (Lupien et al., 2000), but findings are not entirely consistent (Kristenson et al., 2004). Steptoe et al. (2003a) found higher cortisol concentrations in lower-than higher-grade men, but an opposite pattern in women in the Whitehall II Study. However, recently Cohen et al. (2006) demonstrated an inverse relation between SES defined by income and education and stress hormones in humans. Twenty-four-hour urine samples were provided by 193 adults (men and women) for catecholamine determination on each of two days, and seven saliva samples on each of three days, beginning one hour after wake-up, for cortisol analysis. After averaging values across days, lower SES was associated with higher levels of adrenaline and cortisol in a graded fashion independently of race, age, gender and body mass. Noradrenaline followed a similar pattern, but SES differences did not reach statistical significance. These findings support the assumption of SES as a gradient related to allostatic load. Li et al. (2007) investigated salivary cortisol levels in 6335 participants in the 1958 British birth cohort at the age of 45. They found that low socioeconomic position was associated with a larger proportion of extreme post-waking cortisol levels in women and men. They concluded that low SES chronically affects cortisol levels in mid-adult life.

Burke et al. (2005) investigated cortisol responses in 1109 very low-income women and found that women with depressive symptoms had a blunted cortisol response. It has also been found that high psychological well-being is associated with reduced HPA activity at work (Lindfors & Lundberg, 2002; Evans et al., 2007). However, there is considerable variation in stress and health within high- and low-status groups, respectively (Hemström, 2005).

Regardless of social position, women usually report more health problems (e.g. muscle pain, depression, sleep problems, headaches) than men, are on sick leave more often and consume more medication and medical care. Possible reasons for this are discussed in Chapter 10.

Often, low social position is also linked to a below average standard in terms of housing conditions, physical environment, recreational opportunities, and an unhealthier lifestyle, poorer social support, fewer coping alternatives and greater exposure to crime and violence (Marmot, 2004). Each of these factors has been linked to increased health risk. However, clustering of several risk factors is frequent among individuals in low-status positions, whereas high status often involves having access to greater resources and to diverse and more effective coping strategies which are known to enhance health (Marmot, 2004; Cohen *et al.*, 2006). Clustering of risk factors in low-status groups may mean that not only are effects additive, but also they are likely to interact synergistically and thus enhance the health risks. A worker in a low-status job is more likely than a white-collar employee in a high-status job to be a smoker, to have a more unhealthy diet and to be taking no physical exercise off the job, to live in a smaller apartment in an area with more criminality, to have fewer recreational opportunities and less restful scenery around his or her home, and to be exposed to more pollution and noise. This was shown by Evans and Kantrowitz (2002) who found an inverse relationship between SES and a number of environmental risk factors such as exposure to hazardous wastes and toxins, air pollutants, bad water quality, noise, overcrowding, low housing quality and poor neighbourhood conditions.

During recent decades there has been an increasing health gap between west and east European countries, and also between groups within countries. Russia, Ukraine, Belarus and Moldavia have seen declining health and life expectancy since the collapse of the Soviet Union (Vågerö, 2010). In a report from the WHO Task Force on Health System Research Priorities for Equity in Health, Östlin (2004) recommends that highest priority be given to research in five general areas that affect health equity:

1. Important global factors and processes.
2. Specific societal and political structures and relationships.
3. Interrelationships between individual-level factors and social context.
4. Health-care systems.
5. Documenting and disseminating of effective policy interventions.

The WHO Commission on Social Determinants of Health (Marmot, 2008) was formed with the overarching goal of identifying social mechanisms and pathways between social conditions and health and promoting policies and practices that would reduce avoidable global health inequalities with special focus on developing countries. The Commission compiled evidence to form a knowledge base, developed an inventory of policies, and proposed recommendations and health-related policies. The work covered three areas: scientific research, communication and political leadership, and addressed themes such as social gradients, early life, food and nutrition, housing, working conditions and global processes. The Commission report was published in 2008 and forms part of WHO's agenda. The three principles of action (p. 2) are:

1. 'Improve the conditions of daily life – the circumstances in which people are born, grow, live, work and age.' One important measure is to contribute to fair employment and decent work.

2. 'Tackle the inequitable distribution of power, money, and resources – the structural drivers of those conditions of daily life – globally, nationally, and locally.' One important role for governments is to regulate the market and increase market responsibility to ensure that the global economy and the deregulation and liberalisation of the market do not increase health inequity.

3. 'Measure the problem, evaluate action, expand the knowledge base, develop a workforce that is trained in the social determinants of health, and raise public awareness about the social determinants of health.' Monitoring and evaluating changes in social determinants of health and their consequences are important parts of this principle of action.

9 Health Promotion

HEALTH INTERVENTION, STRESS REDUCTION

Individual, organisational and societal conditions all contribute to stress. As a consequence, measures aimed at reducing stress must be introduced at all these levels. Interventions on an individual level are of course important but are often not enough. Interventions on an organisational or societal level are usually more cost-effective as they involve more people. With regard to individual recommendations, such as saying to a person that, in order to reduce stress, 'You must learn how to say no!', 'Just take it easy', 'Don't work too hard', 'Don't rush', 'Don't think about your job outside working hours', 'Make sure you have a good night's sleep' etc., is problematic for several reasons. It is often difficult to follow these recommendations, as their consequences may sometimes induce even more stress. For example, in the caring professions (e.g. nursing, teaching, etc.), it is not possible to say no to a suffering patient or a child in need of help; and if your stress is due to an overwhelming workload, 'just taking it easy' would only make the situation worse. Furthermore, most people want to do a good job and feel bad if they cannot live up to their own, their colleagues' and managers' expectations by carrying out a high quality service. To tell a person under stress how important it is to sleep 8 hours each night is likely to make him or her more worried, and make it even more difficult for him or her to go to sleep.

Individual lifestyle factors such as physical activity, dietary habits, cigarette smoking and alcohol consumption have an important impact on health and are also stress related. Under excessive pressure it is tempting to skip exercise, to eat fast (fatty) food, to smoke more and to drink more alcohol. Stress from work overload can be reduced by trying to replace less important activities with things that make one feel good, as pleasant activities do not tax the individual's resources to the same extent as 'things you have to do'. For example, spending more time on hobbies, listening to music, reading, and interacting with friends and relatives are important for well-being. Because of lack of time, people under occupational stress are less likely to invite friends and relatives for dinner and social interaction. However, social bonds are known to be very important for mental and physical health (Uchino, 2004). Some cultural activities, such as singing, dancing, listening to music and going to the cinema, the theatre, a museum or an art exhibition, have been found to reduce stress levels and improve

The Science of Occupational Health: Stress, Psychobiology and the New World of Work, first edition
By Ulf Lundberg and Cary L. Cooper. Published 2011 by Blackwell Publishing Ltd
© 2011 Ulf Lundberg and Cary L. Cooper

immune functions, provided that these activities are perceived as enjoyable and performed as recreation. Professional singers, dancers, musicians and artists, on the other hand, are from very competitive environments and their striving for perfection exposes them to a lot of stress, which means they need to find other stress-reducing recreations. The responsibility for household chores and childcare at home is usually unevenly divided between men and women, even in dual-career families, as discussed in Chapter 10, causing a higher total workload for women and fewer opportunities for rest and recovery. A more equal division of unpaid work and responsibility would reduce stress in many working women. Improved stress management and relaxation training could also contribute to stress reduction on an individual level.

MANAGING STRESS IN A CHANGING WORKFORCE

Experiences of stress depend to some extent on individual characteristics. Individuals with low self-confidence are at greater risk of developing stress-related symptoms compared with individuals with more realistic views. Being overconfident may also cause problems, such as disappointment and stress, when the individual realises that a situation is beyond their capabilities. It is possible to support individuals and help them to develop methods and resources that increase their ability to intervene and cope with stressful situations.

Cartwright and Cooper (2004) distinguish between primary, secondary and tertiary levels of workplace interventions. For the prevention and management of stress at work, the following three approaches could provide a comprehensive strategic framework: primary prevention (e.g. stress reduction), secondary prevention (e.g. stress management), and tertiary prevention (e.g. employee assistance programmes/workplace counselling).

'Primary prevention' is concerned with taking action to modify or eliminate sources of stress inherent in the work environment, so reducing their negative impact on the individual. The focus of primary interventions is on adapting the environment to 'fit' the individual.

Possible strategies to reduce workplace stress factors include:

- Redesigning the task.
- Redesigning the working environment.
- Establishing flexible work schedules.
- Encouraging participative management.
- Including the employee in career development.
- Analysing work roles and establishing goals.
- Providing social support and response.
- Building cohesive teams.
- Establishing fair employment policies.
- Sharing rewards.

Primary intervention strategies are often a vehicle for culture change. The type of action required by an organisation will vary according to the kinds of stress factors operating. Any intervention, therefore, needs to be guided by prior diagnosis, or a stress audit or risk assessment (such as by ASSET, an organisational stress screening tool: Faragher *et al.*, 2004) to identify the specific factors responsible for employee stress.

'Secondary prevention' is concerned with the prompt detection and management of experienced stress. This can be done by increasing awareness and improving the stress management skills of the individual through training and educative activities. Individual factors can alter or modify the way employees, exposed to workplace stress, perceive and react to their environment. Each individual has his or her own personal stress threshold, which is why some people thrive in a certain setting and others suffer.

Awareness activities and skills training programmes have an important part to play in extending the individual's physical and psychological resources. Such programmes include training in human relations, cognitive coping skills and work/lifestyle modification skills (e.g. time management courses or assertiveness training). The role of secondary prevention is, however, one of damage limitation. Often the consequences of stress are being dealt with, rather than the sources, which may be inherent in the organisation's structure or culture. They are concerned with improving the 'adaptability' of the individual to the environment. Consequently, this type of intervention is often described as the 'band aid' approach. The implicit assumption is that the organisation will continue to be stressful; therefore the individual has to develop and strengthen his or her resistance to that stress.

'Tertiary prevention' is concerned with the treatment, rehabilitation and recovery of individuals who have suffered, or are suffering, from serious ill health as a result of stress (Palmer et al., 2003). Intervention at the tertiary level typically involves provision of counselling services, either by in-house counsellors or outside agencies. These provide counselling, information and/or referral to appropriate treatment and support services. There is evidence to suggest that counselling is effective in improving the psychological well-being of employees and has considerable cost benefits (Palmer et al., 2003; Passmore & Anagnos, 2009). Counselling can be particularly effective in helping employees deal with workplace stress that cannot be changed. It can also help non-work-related stress (e.g. bereavement, marital breakdown, etc.), which tends to spill over into work life.

INDIVIDUAL INTERVENTIONS

As described in Chapter 4, Type A behaviour is a personality-related factor that has been of considerable interest to those studying work–stress–health relationships. Programmes to modify Type A behaviour in healthy individuals have not been very successful. A reason is that this behavioural pattern is encouraged by conditions in the labour market, within organisations and in society in general. Employees who are competitive, productive, job-involved and efficient and who maintain a high work pace are often rewarded by management through better payment and greater career opportunities. Therefore, it is difficult to motivate healthy workers to change their behaviour, as this behaviour pattern is perceived as an important part of their occupational success. However, interventions to reduce Type A behaviour in patients who have already suffered a heart attack have been more successful. Friedman et al. (1986) followed about 1000 post-myocardial infarction patients for 4.5 years to determine whether modification of their Type A (coronary-prone) behaviour would affect their subsequent cardiac morbidity and mortality rates. Participants were randomly assigned either to group cardiac counselling, both group cardiac counselling and Type A behavioural counselling, or a comparison group that did not receive counselling of any kind. Type A behaviour was significantly reduced at the end of the 4.5 year period in 35% of participants given cardiac and Type A behaviour counselling compared with 10% of participants given only cardiac counselling. The cumulative cardiac recurrence rate was significantly less in the group that received both cardiac and Type A counselling (12.9%) than in the group that received cardiac counselling only (21.2%) and in those not receiving any group counselling at all (28.2%). It was concluded that altering Type A behaviour reduces cardiac morbidity and mortality in post-infarction patients. In recent decades, the hostility component of this behaviour pattern has been of particular interest and importance and, consequently, programmes to reduce hostility and manage anger have been developed and have proved successful (Williams & Williams, 1994)

Another individual factor known to be of importance for work-related stress responses is locus of control. High external locus of control means that the employee believes that he or she has very little influence and control over what is happening at work, whereas high internal locus of control means that the employee feels that he or she can influence what is happening to them through their own actions and decisions. External locus of control is associated with more stress at work, and hence, by helping employees to gain more control over their own situation, stress will be reduced. Cognitive behavioural techniques have been developed and found to be particularly efficient in changing people's thinking about how to cope with and respond to various demands.

In addition to personality and cognitive factors, health-promoting interventions also include changes in unhealthy behaviours. Smoking cessation programmes, stimulation of physical exercise, relaxation training and promotion of healthy dietary habits are typical components involved in these programmes. Regular physical exercise has been found to be a particularly important part of health promotion programmes, influencing not only physical fitness and health, but also mental health, for example by reducing depression and anxiety and improving sleep. The role of physical activity for stress and health is presented below.

More extensive intervention programmes should also involve regular health check-ups, health screening, improved health care and family support and care. The effects of single workplace health interventions are usually rather short-lived (Ivancevich & Matteson, 1987) and need to be followed up with boosting and additional interventions. Stress management training programmes can focus on single or multiple factors as described by Cartwright and Whatmore (2005):

1. Stress awareness and education.
2. Relaxation techniques.
3. Cognitive coping strategies.
4. Biofeedback.
5. Meditation.
6. Exercise.
7. Lifestyle advice.
8. Interpersonal skills training.

The aim of individual stress management programmes is to help the employee to gain more control and personal influence over how they handle stressful situations and, consequently, to reduce stress and stress-related health problems. However, the individual cannot influence all conditions at work and depends, to a large extent, on external conditions and demands created on an organisational and societal level. Therefore, individually targeted programmes also need to be complemented by environmental interventions on different levels. Indications of work-related stress problems, which the organisation should act upon, are among others a high or increasing absenteeism, high turnover of staff, poor quality control, reduced efficiency, frequent accidents and conflicts.

HEALTHY WORK

According to established models of occupational stress described in Chapter 4, a reasonable balance between perceived demands and perceived individual resources to handle these demands is necessary for successful coping, optimal performance, well-being and health. Stress typically arises when perceived demands exceed the individual's perceived resources, but occurs also when the demands are far below the individual's capacity. Adequate rewards, feedback and a sense of influence and control are also key factors for healthy work. Uncertainty and insecurity contribute to mental health problems such as stress, anxiety, worry and sleep disorders. Such mental disorders have increased markedly in young people in Europe during the last two decades. For example, Lager and Bremberg (2009) investigated the relationship between national labour trends and young people's mental health in the WHO study, Health Behaviour in School-aged Children, in ten European countries between 1983 and 2005. The countries were Austria, Belgium, Denmark, Finland, Hungary, Norway, Spain, Sweden, Switzerland and the UK. The authors found a very strong relationship between increases in mental health problems among young people and the proportion of people who were not part of the labour force. The correlation between changes in the proportion of 15- to 24-year-olds not part of the labour force and changes in symptoms of feeling low, headache and difficulties going to sleep was 0.92 for girls and 0.77 for boys. This shows that mental problems among young people in Europe are very strongly related to the chances of getting a job.

Decades of stress research have identified a number of occupational health risks but to a large extent researchers have also tried to use this information to define work conditions and individual characteristics that promote health (Karasek & Theorell, 1990; Richter *et al.*, 2007; Cooper *et al.*, 2009; Schnall *et al.*, 2009). Leaders in both the public and private sectors have a very important role in relation to employees' health and well-being at work. A manager has at least three important tasks. One is to keep up with the production demands and see to it that high quality goods and services are produced and delivered on time. A second important task is to encourage and create an organisation that enhances the physical and psychological well-being of its employees. A third task is to be flexible and plan for the future. Under stress, keeping up with the production demands is likely to become the overarching goal, sometimes with negative consequences for the mental health of the employees who have to carry out the actual work tasks. Innovative plans for the future are also likely to be compromised under stressful work conditions.

A manager should listen to the employees, inform and support them and give adequate feedback. Mutual trust between management and workers and being an available and supportive boss will create higher morale in the organisation and stimulate productivity. Managers tend to espouse the view that 'The most valuable resource is our human resource'. What we need is for them to action this rather than just talk about it! Workers should be able to learn about future plans of the organisation, and have a chance to discuss and influence them. An open and engaging leadership style is very important for health and productivity in the organisation. Organisational stress management and prevention programmes are likely to improve mental and physical health, increase productivity and quality, and reduce sickness absence and staff turnover. Interventions to reduce stress should be evaluated from a qualitative as well as a quantitative aspect. A qualitative evaluation can involve focus groups, performance appraisal, informal discussions and interviews. Quantitative measures are productivity and performance data, absenteeism, staff turnover and subjective and physiological stress measures. A number of instruments have been developed for measuring perceived stress at work (job content questionnaire, effort–reward imbalance and stress–energy measures, perceived work stress scale: Faragher *et al.*, 2004), and examples of useful biomarkers of stress are heart rate, blood pressure, blood lipids, blood glucose metabolism (glycated haemoglobin, HbA1c) and stress hormones (Chapter 5).

A comprehensive stress prevention programme would include different levels. Physical health hazards, violence, harassment, bullying and immediate exposure to stress should be reduced or eliminated first; the organisation's ability to identify and deal with stress-related problems should be improved; and individuals suffering from stress-related disorders should receive help to cope with and recover from their problems at work. Around 5% of workers in the 25 EU countries in 2005 reported having experienced some form of violence, bullying or harassment in the workplace in the previous 12-month period (Parent-Thirion *et al.*, 2007).

Adequate and fair rewards in terms of salary, career opportunities and job security are important parts of a job and are positively linked to well-being and health. As differences in health are strongly related to social position, reducing economic and educational differences should be one important societal goal in order to improve health. As described in Chapter 8, the WHO has recently adopted a document on 'Reducing health inequities through action on the social determinants of health' on the basis of recommendations from the Commission on Social Determinants of Health (Marmot, 2008).

As described in Chapters 2 and 3, new forms of work with more flexibility and lack of limitations in terms of time and space, goal-directed work, and access to modern communication technology in terms of mobile phones, email and the internet, make the distinction between work and other parts of life more diffuse. In order to have opportunities for rest and restitution, rules and regulations in society and economic incentives are necessary to help and encourage individuals to reduce stress. Working parents with small children are at particular risk of work overload, and of conflicts between different demands and, in addition, often have insufficient rest and recovery due to disturbed sleep. Therefore, economic and emotional support, counselling and access to high quality day care for children should be prioritised to improve mental and physical health in the workforce.

Findings from research on work-related stress and health should be translated into actions and information that is relevant, valid, useful and understandable for practitioners. Researchers should work closely with the participants to obtain comments and feedback about their applied research results. Researchers need to learn how to communicate their results efficiently to the individuals who are influenced by their findings. For obvious practical, economic and ethical reasons, evaluations of interventions in working life cannot be performed in the same way as the testing of a new drug to treat a disease or an ailment. A double-blind randomised controlled study is usually necessary to provide evidence for the efficacy of a new medicine above the effects of placebo treatment (anticipation effects). Both the patient and the doctor (experimenter) should be unaware of the kind of treatment that is provided, (medication or placebo) in order not to influence and bias the results. This kind of evidence-based research is not possible when evaluating occupational health interventions. Interventions cannot be randomised between employees within a specific work organisation. A control group of employees not going through an intervention or reorganisation has to be found at another workplace. Even if a comparable control group is found, just taking measurements may cause changes, and information may leak out about the ongoing investigation which could influence people's behaviour and health. Furthermore, ongoing changes in society, not controlled by the investigators (such as a financial crisis, a natural disaster and political changes), may have dramatic effects on the participants' work situation and health. For example, in the event of a recession, work sites participating in the evaluation of specific health interventions may have to cut down on personnel or close down completely, which will also influence employees who remain in the study by creating intrinsic insecurity and worry.

However, more 'soft' evaluations are possible. For example, a marked shift in absenteeism, health costs, quality and/or quantity of production after an intervention, compared with a similar company in which no intervention was made, could show the importance of the improvements. Follow-ups over longer periods are usually necessary to identify effects of an intervention, because short-term positive effects which disappear after a while are quite common when health interventions are introduced. A classical example is in the so-called Hawthorne effect, a term coined by Henry Landsberger on the basis of findings from a Western Electric manufacturing facility outside Chicago, the Hawthorne Works, in the 1920s and 1930s. Experiments with higher or lower levels of light showed that any change seemed to improve productivity in the short term. It was assumed that the productivity gain was due to increased motivation among the workers, caused by the interest being shown in them rather than the physical changes at the workplace. The ongoing trend of repeated and more and more frequent reorganisations means that results of long-term investigations are more limited, but examples of successful occupational programmes can be found.

Cooper and Sadri (1991) performed an evaluation of a workplace counselling programme among 250 UK Post Office employees, involving people from shop floor to senior management. Over a one-year period, improvements were found in anxiety and depression levels, somatic symptoms and self-esteem. Sickness absence decreased compared with a matched control group, and the savings for the Post Office were estimated to be about £100 000 over a 6-month period. Nine employee assistance programmes and counselling services were evaluated by Berridge *et al.* (1997) at three different time points: pre-counselling, post-counselling, and 3–6 months after counselling. Comparison was made with an (unmatched) control group of employees and it was found that mental and physical health improved significantly from pre- to post-counselling and there was a significant reduction in both the total number of days absent and the number of absence events. Despite some methodological weaknesses, this is considered one of the most rigorous and extensive outcome studies of UK workplace counselling. McLeod (2001) performed an extensive review of counselling in the workplace, covering reports between 1954 and 2000 involving more than 10 000 clients. It was found that more than 90% of the employees who made use of workplace counselling were highly satisfied with the service. In recent years, there have been very few studies on workplace counselling. The reason for this is not clear, but the complexity of this kind of research in a rapidly changing work environment may be one reason and suspicion and fear on the part of stakeholders could be another.

Knapp (2009) performed a systematic review of studies published between 1997 and 2007 on the effects of workplace health promotion intervention on depression and anxiety symptoms. Twenty-two studies comprising 3409 employees met the inclusion criteria. The general result showed that a broad range of health promotion interventions were effective in reducing symptoms of depression and anxiety among employees, although the effects were rather small. Wahlstedt and co-workers (Wahlstedt & Edling 1997; Wahlstedt *et al.*, 2000) followed 100 postal workers for 12 months and found that improvements in the work organisation reduced MSD and gastrointestinal and sleep problems and decreased sick leave and staff turnover.

PricewaterhouseCoopers (2008) carried out an evaluation of 55 wellness programmes in the UK, exploring the impact of these on a number of outcome factors (i.e. sickness absence, employee satisfaction, etc.) in an effort to assess the business case for well-being interventions. They found that over all the 55 programmes there was an average decline of 45% in sickness absence, 18% in staff turnover and 16% in accidents and injuries at work, and a 4% increase in employee satisfaction. There was also a fall of 9% in resource allocation, an 8% improvement in company profile, an 8% increase in productivity, an 8% improvement in health and welfare, a 7% decline in health and other insurance claims and a 4% increase in competitiveness and profitability. The study also highlighted the direct cost savings of several of the case-study companies, for example, a financial services company of 3000 employees showed the following improvements after a stress management, counselling and healthy living programme: an 80% decrease in stress absence, a 20% decrease in staff turnover, a 1% increase in productivity and a 5% decrease in smokers, for an overall absence-related cost saving of just over £250 000 in a year.

MENTAL CAPITAL AND WELL-BEING

The findings from the UK Government's Foresight Project on Mental Capital and Well-being (Fig. 9.1) was a landmark report on what enhances and depletes an individual's mental capital through life or debits or credits their well-being, metaphorically a 'bank account of the mind'. This project involved more than 400 experts and stakeholders from different disciplines in 16 countries. The aim was to address the challenges of depression, dementia, learning

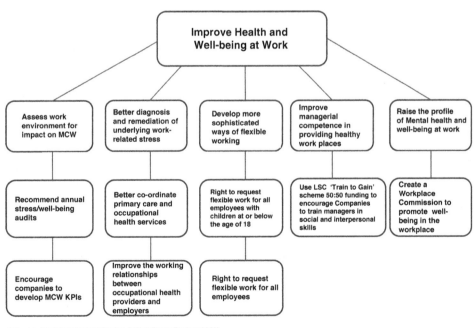

(Source: Foresight Mental Capital & Well-Being Project 2008)

Fig. 9.1   Interventions suggested by the Foresight MCW Project for the Improvement of Health and Well-being at Work.

difficulties and mental ill-health. The project was focused on two main aspects: mental capital and mental well-being.

Mental capital includes both cognitive and emotional resources relevant for the individual's ability to contribute to society and to experience a high quality of life. *Mental well-being* refers to the individuals' ability to develop their potential, work productively and creatively, build strong and positive relationships with others and contribute to their community. The project examined peer-reviewed papers to understand the latest evidence and to identify possible ways of moving forward with regard to childhood development, mental health and well-being at work, and making the most of cognitive resources in older age. The following key findings were emphasised:

1. The importance of boosting brain power in the young and adults in order to improve mental capital through different types of intervention.
2. Based on biomarkers early in life, science can reveal learning difficulties.
3. Early detection of mental disorders is essential. There is great potential for improving diagnosis and treatment and to address social risk factors.
4. Learning must continue throughout life as this can have a direct effect on mental health and well-being across all age groups.
5. Changing needs in changing workplaces have to be identified in order to improve the mental capital of economies and societies.

The authors (Beddington *et al.*, 2008) point out the costs of not acting on the basis of these findings. For example, learning difficulties affect up to 10% of children and can also lead to behavioural problems, social exclusion, unemployment and crime. Mental ill-health is a very widespread problem and depression is the leading global cause of years lived with disability. The annual costs of mental illness in England alone are about $77 billion. With an ageing population, the costs of mental illness are expected to rise markedly in the future as the elderly population of over 65s is likely to double and of over 80s to treble over the next 40 years in most developed countries, and the cost of dementia to at least treble during that period. Early interventions according to the report are essential for a beneficial development.

One of the major strands of the work was 'work and well-being', a number of science reviews emphasising the main sources of workplace stress as highlighted by Cooper *et al.* (2009). These authors identified seven major sources of stress associated with a lack of mental well-being at work: an autocratic or bullying management style, a perceived lack of control or involvement in decision-making by employees, a marked lack of skill utilisation and variety, excessive workloads, the lack of clarity of one's role, poor working relationships between work colleagues, the lack of social support at work, and long working hours leading to lack of work–life balance.

For any one individual a combination of these factors, together with the personality and coping strategies of the individual, will lead to either positive or negative well-being outcomes. Of course the context is also important, particularly at times of economic crisis and increasing job insecurity, a significant move to presenteeism (where people feel they have to work longer hours to be seen to be present at work, even if they have little to do!), fewer people doing more work (to keep the labour costs down), and a more robust if not controlling management style to meet the bottom-line demands of top management.

In addition to the Foresight findings, much research (e.g. Rayner *et al.*, 2002; Robertson & Flint-Taylor, 2009) has found that an autocratic, bullying management style can adversely affect not only an individual's health but also people's performance. A management style that on the other hand provides individuals with some locus of control and autonomy is likely to be more effective and enhance one's mental capital and well-being (Siegrist, 2008). Excessive workloads have also been found to relate to stress and ill-health, particularly in the context of being unable to control aspects of the job. For example, numerous studies have been carried out using Karasek's (1979) job Demand–Control model, and have found that people who have high demand and low control show major stress-related outcomes (Cartwright & Cooper, 2009). In addition to the way a person is managed as regards his/her control over the job and the demands on them, the hours worked and their impact on health and family are another major source of depleted mental capital and well-being. There is extensive research that shows that long working hours can damage one's health (Burke & Cooper, 2008), and that flexible working arrangements can alleviate the stress and enhance job satisfaction, health and family relationships (Spector *et al.*, 2007).

INTERVENTIONS AND POLICIES

A number of possible interventions and policies were developed following the Foresight project. A team of economists was given the task of carrying out cost–benefit analyses of a number of these possible interventions (where possible and practicable), and these were highlighted in the final report (Cooper *et al.*, 2009).

First, the evidence suggested that 'how' people manage other people at work, whether in the private or public sector, is critical not only to their effective performance, but also to their health and well-being. This requires better social and interpersonal skills among managers, which means enhanced training to emphasise the 'people management' skills and competences and not just the technical parts of their job (i.e. marketing, operational management, human resources policies/law, etc.).

Secondly, most organisations are so fast moving and focused on immediate returns that they lose touch with their employees' concerns and issues. One way to track the health and well-being aspects of work is to engage in regular well-being or stress audits screening through psychometric measures already available, such as ASSET (Faragher *et al.*, 2004). The evidence is that performing regular audits by collecting the views (anonymously) of employees on how they perceive their job, their organisation, their management, etc., and then systematically intervening to deal with the problems highlighted, can have a major impact on reducing stress, sickness absence and turnover, and enhancing mental well-being. This is currently 'best practice' in a small number of global companies and larger public-sector bodies, but not very prevalent in most small to medium-sized businesses or public-sector organisations (Dewe *et al.*, 2010).

Thirdly, the evidence shows that working long hours can damage people's mental well-being, particularly at a time when the average family is a two-earner family. Long hours can adversely affect health, performance and family relationships (Burke & Cooper, 2008). The Foresight Report (Cooper *et al.*, 2009) suggests that one answer to this is 'flexible working arrangements', or at least 'the right to request' these arrangements for all employees, not just the ones with children. Indeed, another stream of the Foresight project found that by 2070 there would be twice the number of 65-year-olds (around 21 million) and three times the number of 80-year-olds (nearly 10 million) in the UK. The issue of elder care will therefore become an even greater reality than today. In addition, the implications of this demographic trend for the health and well-being of the elderly themselves are quite profound, with evidence suggesting that the longer people work, if they choose to do so, whether in paid employment or in a volunteering capacity, the less likely they are to suffer from dementia and other 'cognitive declining' conditions. The human costs are high, but so also are the enormous costs to society: Foresight estimated that by 2038 the number of people suffering from dementia will double from 1.4 million, and the costs of care and treatment will treble from £17 billion to £50 billion per annum.

PHYSICALLY RISKY JOBS

Work conditions that are known to be associated with increased health risks, such as repetitive assembly work and tasks combining heavy physical work and mental stress, should, of course, as far as possible be eliminated or improved. However, despite extensive ergonomic and organisational improvements, certain work tasks associated with health risks cannot be completely abolished. For example, in caring jobs such as nursing, it is often necessary to lift patients, and unexpected events may happen that make it essential to act quickly without thinking about optimal ergonomic recommendations, for instance if a patient loses balance or consciousness and is about to fall. Police officers and firefighters are workers who are frequently exposed to physical and mental health risks in their jobs. Long-term exposure to monotonous work, static load and repetitive movements among assembly workers, cashiers, data entry workers and workers at call centres is associated with health problems such as neck, shoulder and back pain. The health risks increase with the time of exposure, and individuals who tend to stay longer in such jobs are often women. This could partly explain why women develop more health problems compared with men, for example neck and shoulder pain. Men more often than women move to other work tasks and more senior positions in the organisation after a shorter period in such jobs, and thus are less exposed to long-term, unhealthy, repetitive work and static load conditions. Similar mechanisms (staying longer in the same risky job) may explain why immigrants often develop more health problems than other workers. By reducing the time the worker is exposed to such conditions before symptoms start to appear, and by providing time for rest, recovery and recuperation, the health risks can be limited. One way to reduce the amount of exposure to risky work conditions that it has not been possible to eliminate completely is to offer each worker an individual plan of development and variation that enables him or her to replace risky work tasks after a period of time by more healthy and hopefully more stimulating work. This is likely to bring about greater job involvement, more satisfaction and better health. Such a plan needs to be followed up and rescheduled on an annual basis.

POSITIVE PSYCHOLOGY

Most research has focused on negative psychosocial factors and occupational health risks, and very little on health promotion, the individual and occupational factors contributing to good health. Why do some workers stay healthy and live longer than others? In recent years, interest in such 'salutogenic' factors has grown. To a large extent good health can be defined by the experience of being healthy, and a number of studies have shown that subjective good health ratings predict morbidity as well as mortality. Individuals reporting that they have very good subjective health have fewer symptoms and live longer than individuals who report that they have poor subjective health (Ferraro & Su, 2000; Kyffin et al., 2004). Self-reports even seem to have greater predictive value than physician-evaluated morbidity (Ferraro & Su, 2000).

In 1979, Aaron Antonovsky, who was active at Ben Gurion University in Israel, formulated a theory of sense of coherence, measuring three psychological dimensions of importance for being in control of the environment: comprehensibility, manageability, and meaningfulness. He found that individuals with a strong sense of coherence had a better chance of surviving and staying healthy under stressful conditions. 'Comprehensibility' is a belief that events are ordered, consistent and structured and a sense that one can understand what is happening in life and predict what will happen in the future. 'Manageability' is a belief that one has the necessary resources to cope with life events. 'Meaningfulness' is a belief that life makes sense and that things are interesting and create satisfaction in life. A number of studies have shown that high sense of coherence is associated with positive health outcomes (review by Eriksson & Lindström, 2005). Surtees *et al.* (2003, 2006) investigated the relationship between a strong sense of coherence and mortality in a prospective study of more than 20 000 individuals (41–80 years) for 6 years and found that a strong sense of coherence was associated with a 30% reduction in all-cause mortality and cardiovascular and cancer mortality, independent of age, sex and prevalent chronic disease. High sense of coherence has also been associated with lower allostatic load in middle-aged women (Lindfors *et al.*, 2006).

More recently, Carol Ryff and colleagues (e.g. Ryff & Singer, 1998) have constructed a scale (see Table 9.1) that measures psychological well-being based on psychological factors that contribute to positive feelings and health. This scale consists of six dimensions: autonomy, environmental mastery, personal growth, positive relations with others, purpose in life, and self-acceptance. Individuals with high scores on this scale have been found to be healthier and live longer than others and to have a 'buffer' against negative life events. Even under stressful conditions with serious life events, individuals who are high in psychological well-being seem to have resources that help them to cope and stay healthy. Ryff has a broader definition of positive psychology than Antonovsky, but her scale includes dimensions that overlap with the concept of sense of coherence. Ryff has investigated how psychological well-being varies with age, gender and socioeconomic status (e.g. Ryff & Singer, 1998). Early life experiences have proved to be of particular importance for adult psychological well-being. Individuals with a warm, safe and stimulating childhood are more

Table 9.1 Examples of items from the Ryff Psychological Well–being Scale

Autonomy	I have confidence in my opinions even if they are contrary to the general consensus. Being happy with myself is more important than having others approve of me.
Environmental mastery	I am quite good at managing the many responsibilities of my daily life. I generally do a good job of taking care of my personal finances and affairs.
Personal growth	I think it is important to have new experiences that challenge how you think about the world. I have the sense that I have developed a lot as a person over time.
Positive relations with others	Most people see me as loving and affectionate. I enjoy personal and mutual conversations with family members or friends.
Purpose in life	I am an active person in carrying out the plans I set for myself. I enjoy making plans for the future and working to make them a reality.
Self-acceptance	The past had its ups and downs, but in general I wouldn't want to change it. When I compare myself with friends and acquaintances, it makes me feel good about who I am.

likely to express a high level of psychological well-being as adults. This is consistent with the animal experiments of Meaney and his colleagues which showed that rat mother–pup interaction early in life determines the animal's ability to deal successfully with life events as an adult. In humans it is likely that not only childhood experiences but also conditions later in life, such as education, family and occupation, are of importance for psychological well-being.

As described in Chapter 6, extensive research has revealed psychobiological mechanisms linking negative stress experiences to health problems, and several models for occupational stress–health relationships have been formulated (Demand–Control, ERI). With regard to salutogenic factors, however, research on the biological underpinning of positive psychology and biomarkers of good health is still limited. One reason for this is that health has usually been defined as the absence of medical symptoms and biological parameters outside the normal range. A healthy person is therefore an individual without health complaints and with normal levels of blood pressure, glucose and blood lipids, normal renal function and electrocardiogram, etc. However, in 1948 the WHO defined health as 'a state of complete physical, mental and social well-being and not merely the absence of disease or infirmity'.

Another salutogenetic concept, which has reached considerable popularity in recent years, is 'mindfulness'. This is a state of consciousness characterised by an ongoing calm awareness of and attention to the stream of internal and external experiences. It involves a heightened awareness of sensory stimuli (noticing your breathing, feeling the sensations of your body, etc.) and being 'in the now'. Scientific support for the positive effects of mindfulness-based stress-reduction interventions for mental and emotional health is still limited, but some recent studies are promising. Nykliček and Kuijpers (2008) compared the effects of a mindfulness-based stress-reduction (MBSR) intervention on a waiting-list control condition in a randomised controlled trial with 40 women and 20 men. Results showed that, compared with the control group, the intervention resulted in significantly stronger reductions of perceived stress and vital exhaustion and stronger elevations of positive affect, quality of life, and mindfulness. It was concluded that increased mindfulness may, at least partly, mediate the positive effects of MBSR intervention. Kimbrough *et al.* (2010) exposed 27 adult survivors of childhood sexual abuse to 8-week MBSR. Statistically significant improvements were observed in depressive symptoms, post-traumatic stress disorder (PTSD), anxiety and mindfulness.

One line of salutogenic research is the investigation of biological factors that contribute to the reduction of pain and stress, and which induce a sense of harmony, calmness and relaxation. In a series of studies Kerstin Uvnäs-Moberg at the Karolinska Institute in Sweden and her colleagues have focused on the role of oxytocin as an 'anti-stress hormone' contributing to well-being, social interaction, growth and healing (Uvnäs-Moberg & Petterson, 2005). Oxytocin is a hormone excreted during breast-feeding that stimulates lactation and social and maternal behaviour, and induces a feeling of harmony and relaxation. It is also secreted during childbirth and stimulates contractions during labour and contributes to a stronger attachment between mother and child (Jonas, 2009). Oxytocin is secreted by men too, and reduces pain sensitivity, promotes weight gain and growth and attenuates cortisol responses to mental stress. Massage, skin-to-skin contact and stroking increase oxytocin secretion and induce feelings of well-being.

In addition to oxytocin, endogenous endorphins are of interest as biomarkers of health and well-being. Endorphins are natural pain relievers and induce a sense of well-being. These peptide hormones are produced in response to exercise, excitement and orgasm, and also in response to stress and pain.

RESTORATIVE ENVIRONMENTS AND RECREATION

Natural scenery has a stress-reducing effect compared with exposure to an urban environment dominated by stressed people, concrete buildings, noise, pollution and traffic. A possible explanation for this is that green areas with trees, flowers, lawns, water and birds do not tax one's 'executive mental functions' to the same extent as the urban environment. Focused attention in an urban noisy and densely populated area needs active suppression of irrelevant signals from the environment (top–bottom control), whereas enjoying natural scenery needs no effort and does not tax one's executive functions (bottom–top stimulation).

'Executive functioning' involves a number of cognitive factors related to health, such as maintenance and change of health behaviour, stress regulation and management of chronic illness (Williams & Thayer, 2009). Successful programmes leading to weight loss, smoking cessation, and adherence to medical regimens depend on executive functioning. Executive functioning has also been linked to brain function, prefrontal neural function in particular, which is reflected in heart rate variability (HRV). Decreased HRV is a risk factor for heart disease and stroke (Thayer & Lane, 2007). Executive functioning thus has an important role in stress regulation. Deficits in executive functioning have been associated with diabetes, obesity, hypertension, vascular and lung disease, and HIV/AIDS, and executive functioning is central to the processing of pain and emotional signals (Williams & Thayer, 2009). Health problems are likely to lead to further decrements in executive functioning. Physical exercise, stress regulation interventions and cognitive behaviour therapy are factors assumed to improve executive functioning. These relationships emphasise the importance of integrating brain functions (mind), physiology and behaviour in understanding, prevention and treatment of work-related health problems.

Terry Hartig, an American researcher active at Uppsala University, Sweden, has performed a series of studies on how people recover from ordinary psychological wear-and-tear, with specific interest in the places available to people for restoration. In field experiments he has compared the emotional, cognitive, and physiological changes in young adults who walked in either a nature reserve or some urban setting, to test theories about how environments may promote or constrain restoration. In summary, his research supports the notion that green environments, trees and plants promote restoration from work stress and contribute to well-being, health and performance (Hartig, 2008). His aim was to provide information that helped people to maintain and sustain their mental and physical health by reducing demands and promoting restoration possibilities.

The role of restorative activities for depressive symptoms was investigated in nationally aggregated data from Sweden between 1991 and 1998 (Hartig et al., 2007). Most Swedes have their summer holidays in July, and Hartig and colleagues related the temperature in July to the dispensation of antidepressant medication. The assumption that low mean temperature in July was related to increased dispensation of antidepressants (selective serotonin reuptake inhibitors, SSRIs) was confirmed, which indicates that Swedish people are more depressed when the temperature is low and constrains their possibilities for outdoor restorative activities. In addition, Hartig and Fransson (2009) investigated the role of a leisure home for early retirement in 42 588 adults in high-density Swedish urban municipalities. It was found that access to a leisure home reduced the risk of early retirement from work for men, but not for women. The reason for this gender difference is not clear, but could be due to women's greater responsibilities for unpaid work at home, which may be even more demanding in a leisure home with few modern facilities (no running water, no WC, no washing machine or dishwasher, etc.). Because of traditional sex-role patterns in terms of domestic work, living in a leisure home may not offer the same possibilities for women to engage in restorative activities as it does for men.

Recently, Pressman *et al.* (2009) investigated the relationship between enjoyable leisure activities and psychological and physiological factors in 1399 individuals. Participating in more enjoyable leisure activities (time alone and time unwinding, visiting and being with others, doing fun things with others, vacation, hobbies, etc.) was associated with lower levels of depression and negative affect, lower blood pressure, cortisol, waist circumference and BMI, and better physical function.

As 'mentally induced' muscle tension may also keep muscle fibres active during non-work conditions (Chapter 6) and hence increase the risk of developing MSD, it is important to facilitate employee breaks at work to enable them to unwind and relax during the day and at the end of the working day. Veiersted *et al.* (1993) followed a group of healthy female workers starting a new, repetitive job by measurements of muscular activity (trapezius EMG) during work and during breaks at work. The workers were followed for a year, and at the end of the year about half of the women had contracted neck and shoulder pain (trapezius myalgia). It was found that women who contracted myalgia had significantly more muscle activity during breaks at work compared with women who remained healthy. This is consistent with the Cinderella Hypothesis (Chapter 6), and shows that the ability to relax during breaks at work decreases the risk of musculoskeletal pain syndromes.

In addition to sleep, other forms of rest are necessary for optimal performance, health and well-being (Kuijper *et al.*, 1998). Short periods of rest are necessary for keeping attention at an adequate level, for example when listening to a lecture. Relaxation is also of importance for digestion. Consequently, proper time for having lunch and dinner is important for restoration and health. During activity, catabolic processes are prioritised, which means that processes related to digestion and growth are reduced. Longer periods of rest are necessary in the evening, both for digestion of food at dinner, but also for unwinding before sleep. In sedentary work, time off to take a short walk in the middle of the day and after working hours is also important to promote health, and will have positive effects on performance. Regular moderate physical exercise reduces stress and improves immune function, and, as described above, stimulates the production of new brain cells in the hippocampus. However, physical exercise should not be performed just before going to bed, as bodily arousal from physical activity interferes with sleep onset. More on the role of physical activity is presented below.

The weekend is important for the opportunities it provides to perform non-work-related physical activity and to participate in other forms of recreation (hobbies, social interaction, etc.). Even longer periods of recreation, such as a vacation lasting 3–4 weeks, are of importance for health. In some stressful jobs, this is the only period when the employee is able to relax entirely from work, as it can take a week or more to mentally unwind completely from work. Responding to emails and telephone calls during this period may disrupt this deactivation of the physiological stress systems. Studies (e.g. Johansson & Aronsson, 1984) have shown that activity in the central stress systems is reduced during vacation, and that individuals respond more adequately to challenges after vacation than before. A low arousal level is also important for reflection and problem solving, and for being able to be creative and develop new ideas. This means that the first weeks at work after vacation could be a period when employees are particularly creative. In view of the animal study mentioned in Chapter 6, showing that chronic stress causes a shift towards using habitual strategies rather than finding new adequate ways to solve problems, vacation is likely to be important for creative productivity.

Continuous access to email, mobile phones and the internet and a high degree of overcommitment may tempt people also to work during periods meant for relaxation and recovery. Modern communication techniques, combined with expectations from colleagues and the employer that one should be available to respond at any time, may thus interfere with important anabolic processes. However, worrying over what is happening at the job and the accumulation of emails when you are on vacation may be just as stressful, or even worse than checking your email on a regular basis. Under such circumstances, a plan for when to keep in contact with work could be helpful. For example, one solution is that the employee, in agreement with the employer, checks his or her emails once a week during vacation, and gets compensation for that in terms of extra holidays during another part of the year. In more flexible jobs, such as an owner of a business enterprise, work as a freelance journalist or a consultant, being completely detached from work for several weeks is often not possible if one wants to stay in business. However, a similar arrangement to keep in contact with business on specific days during vacation is preferable compared with being available 24–7!

In conclusion, enough time for rest, recovery and recreation are key factors for adequate functioning of important bodily processes and for optimal performance. The worker's ability to influence his or her balance between work, family, recreation and rest is of significant importance for long-term well-being, health and performance.

SLEEP

Sleep is the most important form of rest and recovery, and disturbed sleep is one of the most common complaints among people. Daily human life usually follows a 24-hour rhythm, with activity during the day and sleep during the night. A number of biological functions also follow this circadian rhythm, such as body temperature, endocrine excretion, metabolism and cerebral functions. During sleep deprivation many biological functions continue to vary according to the 24-hour rhythm. For example, adrenaline levels continue to vary in a sinusoidal fashion (peak level in the middle of the day and nadir during the night) after 2–3 days of sleep deprivation. Reversing sleep–wake patterns by staying awake during the night and sleeping during the day will in about a week reverse the biological rhythms. Travelling east- and westwards over time zones will have a similar effect. A slow phase shift of 1–2 hours a day will not have any noticeable effects on performance, and biological systems adapt successively, but rapid shifts, for example from transatlantic flights, will cause the biological and mental disturbances usually described as jet lag.

Sleep is controlled by the suprachiasmatic nuclei of the CNS, and melatonin produced by the pineal gland regulates the sleep–wake cycle by causing drowsiness and lowering the body temperature. During sleep, a number of anabolic processes are active and melatonin secretion peaks. The secretion of sex and growth hormones increases, the immune system is strengthened, memories are consolidated and healing processes are stimulated. According to recent findings reported by Miller (2009), sleep also seems to have an important role in resetting overstimulated synapses after a day of neural activity. As described above, individuals regularly sleeping 7–8 hours a day are more resistant to stress-related disorders and infections (Cohen *et al.*, 2009) and to muscular disorders (Canivet *et al.*, 2008). Experimental studies, where the amount of sleep has been reduced from the normal 8 hours to 6 or 4 hours, show pronounced effects on bodily processes and increased risk of overweight, Type 2 diabetes and increased stress sensitivity (e.g. Spiegel *et al.*, 2005). Healthy young adults who are getting an average of about 5 hours of sleep a night must secrete 30% more insulin than other adults to achieve a normal glucose curve.

An individual's work pattern can be an important determinant of sleep problems as a large part of the working population has irregular work hours. Regular shift work, with two or three shifts, is common, and by rotating 8-hour shifts between weeks the biological rhythms are disturbed and workers have to adjust their diurnal sleep–wake rhythm every week. This usually results in sleep problems and feelings of sleepiness, and is associated with lack of vigour and energy during active work and may increase the occurrence of errors and accidents. Light exposure contributes to the normal circadian rhythms, and therefore it is difficult to stay alert during night work and difficult to go to sleep in daylight. Even permanent night work causes disturbed biological rhythms and sleeping problems because of the effects of light and noise during the day, and the fact that even permanent night workers tend to change their sleep pattern during the weekend for social and family reasons. Sleepiness and lack of alertness are particularly pronounced during night work, when the biological rhythms (low adrenaline, high melatonin) induce sleepiness. This can explain why traffic accidents peak during night hours. The only way to counteract these effects is to provide time for sleep and rest. Air crews flying over several time zones in an east- and westwards direction are also exposed to shift work and in addition to changes in external light/dark cycles. Napping, for example for 30 minutes, is a common way to reduce sleepiness and increase performance among workers on the night shift and among air crews flying over several time zones. Exposure to intensely bright light also increases alertness and performance during night work.

Frost *et al.* (2009) performed a systematic review of studies on the relative risk of ischaemic heart disease in relation to shift work and found a weak causal relation. In a longitudinal study, Suwazono *et al.* (2008) compared the effect of alternating shift work and day work on body mass index in about 7000 Japanese male workers and found that alternating shift work was an independent risk factor for weight gain. In a recent special issue of *Scandinavian Journal of Work, Environment & Health*, Härmä and Kecklund (2010) concluded that shift work, via sleep problems and sleepiness, has a great number of detrimental health consequences, such as safety risks, heart disease, Type 2 diabetes, rheumatoid arthritis, mental health problems and probably peptic ulcers, gastrointestinal symptoms and breast cancer (Parent-Thirion *et al.*, 2007).

PHYSICAL ACTIVITY

'Physical activity' includes all movements of the body produced by skeletal muscles which use energy. Exercise and physical training influence the body by a disturbance of homeostasis. During rest and recovery, homeostasis is restored and the body adapts to the exercise by increasing its functional capacity. Successive training, with proper periods for recovery, is followed by successive increases in capacity and improved performance. Physical exercise has proved to be health promoting, and reduces stress and mental health problems (e.g. depression), pain, the metabolic syndrome and the risk of CHD and improves immune functions. The importance of physical exercise for stress tolerance has been documented in several studies (van Doornen & de Geus, 1989; Nieman, 1998). Regular walking for 30 minutes a day seems to be sufficient to achieve positive effects (Lee *et al.*, 2000). Physical activity has also been found to reduce depressive symptoms (Penninx *et al.*, 2002), to reduce insulin resistance in overweight individuals (Tuomilehto *et al.*, 2001) and to have beneficial effects on fibromyalgia patients (Richards & Scott, 2002). Physical activity is also of importance for rehabilitation from stroke, and in neural and lung diseases. The importance of physical exercise increases with age, as elderly individuals have less physical 'overcapacity' and, hence, will gain more by improving their physical strength and aerobic capacity. Physical activity is often included as an important part of most health intervention programmes, and often recommended by doctors to individual patients.

Blumenthal *et al.* (2005) compared the effect of two behavioural programmes, aerobic exercise training and stress management training, with routine medical care on psychosocial functioning and markers of cardiovascular risk in 134 patients with ischaemic heart disease (92 male and 42 female aged 40–84 years). Patients in the exercise and stress management groups obtained lower depression scores and reduced distress, had smaller reductions in left ventricular ejection fraction during mental stress testing, and had greater improvements in flow-mediated dilation and significant increases in heart rate variability. It was concluded that exercise and stress management training reduced emotional distress and improved markers of cardiovascular risk more than the usual medical care alone for patients with stable ischaemic heart disease.

In a recent worksite health intervention (von Thiele Schwarz *et al.*, 2008), six workplaces with 177 women employed in dentistry were randomised to one of three conditions: (1) 2.5 hours of weekly mandatory physical exercise, (2) 2.5 hours' reduction of full-time weekly work hours, and (3) no change in working conditions at all. The participants retained their normal salary during the intervention period. Measurements including biomarkers of stress and self-ratings were obtained before intervention, after 6 months and after 12 months. Physical exercise increased in all three groups, but most in the group performing physical activity during working hours. Effects on biomarkers were small, but glucose levels and upper-extremity disorders decreased significantly in the exercise group whereas waist–hip ratio increased in the group with reduced working hours. It was concluded that the effects of this short-term intervention were rather small, but that physical exercise during working hours was more effective than just reducing working hours. It is possible that a longer follow-up would have given more pronounced differences between the three conditions. Despite the reduction in working hours (2.5 hours in two of the groups), productivity (number of patients treated) did not change, which indicates that performance efficiency increased.

The importance of physical exercise has also been demonstrated in many other studies (Grønningsæter *et al.*, 1992; Whatmore *et al.*, 1999), which consistently show that, from a health perspective, regular moderate physical exercise is to be preferred compared with excessive exercise or no exercise at all. Brisk walking 30 minutes a day, or similar whole-body exercise (jogging, swimming) five times a week, seems to give optimal positive health effects and is at the same time associated with low risk of injury.

10   Gender Differences

SYMPTOMS, HEALTH AND LIFE EXPECTANCY

Women generally report more health problems than do men. Examples are muscular pains, sleep problems, mood disturbances, chronic fatigue, burnout syndromes, fibromyalgia and headaches. Women also seek medical care and are absent from work more often than men and use more medication. In contrast, women tend to live longer than men, which sometimes has been considered a paradox: 'Women are sicker but men die quicker' (Verbrugge & Wingard, 1987). This 'paradox' can be explained by the fact that the symptoms that women report are usually non-fatal and therefore have little effect on their life expectancy. As described below, men tend to die earlier than women for other reasons. Seeking medical care, the more frequent use of medication, reporting symptoms and being absent from work are factors often considered as signs of illness, but could instead be considered as protective factors and partly explain women's longer life expectancy. By paying attention to symptoms, seeking medical care and using medication to treat a disease or an ailment and being absent from work when ill, women may protect themselves against more serious life-threatening disorders.

Although women generally live longer than men, gender differences in life expectancy vary considerably between social and cultural groups, countries, and over time. In Western Europe and North America, women live on average 3–4 years longer than do men. Life expectancy is increasing in almost all countries in both women and men, but somewhat more for men, and today men live about as long as women did 15–20 years ago. The most pronounced sex difference in longevity can be found in Russia, where life expectancy declined after the collapse of the Soviet Union: today Russian women live more than ten years longer than men. As mentioned earlier, differences in lifespan within countries are strongly related to SES in women and men. This means that sex differences, like SES differences in life expectancy, are influenced by environmental and behavioural factors.

Possible explanations for men's somewhat shorter life expectancy may be lifestyle, work conditions, behaviour and cardiovascular disorders. Men started to smoke cigarettes before women did and thus have been smoking for a longer period of time. As cigarette smoking is one of the most important risk factors for myocardial infarction (Yusuf *et al.*, 2004), this

The Science of Occupational Health: Stress, Psychobiology and the New World of Work, first edition
By Ulf Lundberg and Cary L. Cooper. Published 2011 by Blackwell Publishing Ltd
© 2011 Ulf Lundberg and Cary L. Cooper

has probably contributed to gender differences in heart attacks in the working population. Lung cancer and chronic obstructive lung disease, most often due to cigarette smoking, have also been a more common reason for premature death in men compared with women. Cigarette smoking among women has increased at the same time as it has decreased among men. As a consequence, lung cancer is decreasing among men and increasing among women. Today, death due to lung cancer in women in the USA is more common than death due to breast cancer, and a similar increase in lung cancer deaths in women can be seen in Europe.

With regard to other health-related lifestyle factors, which may contribute to gender differences in life expectancy, men usually have more unhealthy dietary habits than women (Dynesen *et al.*, 2003), and women more often than men perform physical exercise for health reasons (Meyer *et al.*, 2004). As an unhealthy diet and lack of physical exercise are related to cardiovascular disease, these gender differences may contribute to a higher prevalence of cardiovascular disorders among working men.

Men are more often than women exposed to fatal accidents at work. One reason is that men more often work in hazardous jobs, such as police officers, firefighters, soldiers and coal mine workers, but also because men expose themselves to greater risks than women and more often cause fatal accidents, including traffic accidents. Men are more likely to take chances, fail to use protective means (seat belts, helmets) and to follow instructions on how to handle dangerous equipment. Worldwide, road traffic injuries are the second leading cause of death among those aged 15–44 years, and men are involved in accidents more often than women.

Men are also more likely to commit suicide (Hawton, 2000) compared with women, although women more often attempt to commit suicide. The reason for these gender differences is not known, but could be because men select more 'efficient' ways to kill themselves (hanging, breathing vehicle exhaust gas, asphyxiation, firearms and jumping in front of trains) compared with women (self-poisoning, cutting blood vessels), or that women's attempts are not always meant to cause death. It is sometimes difficult to know how serious suicide attempts are and how to classify certain deaths, such as a person being killed after driving a car into a tree or drowning when alone. Statistics from different countries are not always comparable because of social, cultural and religious bias, but it is consistently found that about twice as many men compared with women commit suicide.

Cardiovascular disorders (CVD), such as myocardial infarction and stroke, afflict both women and men. About half of the population in industrialised countries, men as well as women, eventually die because of CVD. However, heart attacks occur earlier in life in men than in women. In the working population, myocardial infarctions are 4–5 times as frequent in men as in women. After menopause at the age of around 50, when the production of oestrogen ceases, the incidence of CVD starts to increase in women. This indicates that natural oestrogen production has a protective role against CVD in women, whereas the positive effects of oestrogen replacement therapy after menopause on coronary heart disease risk are more uncertain (Petitti, 2009).

There are significant differences between men and women in survival following a heart attack. About 40% of women who have heart attacks die within a year compared with about 25% of men (Chou *et al.*, 2007). One possible reason for this difference is that women tend to get heart disease about 10 years later in life than men, when they are older and generally more vulnerable. Furthermore, most research on CVD has been performed on men, and women's symptoms when having a heart attack seem to differ somewhat from those of men and therefore a heart attack is more difficult to diagnose.

Research has shown that women may not be diagnosed as early as men, and also that women with heart disease are treated less aggressively. Diabetes and high LDL cholesterol are risk factors for CVD. Chou *et al.* (2007) found that women with diabetes were 19% less likely than men to have their LDL cholesterol controlled, and women with a history of CVD were 28% less likely than men to have their LDL cholesterol controlled. According to a study of cholesterol management of 243 primary care patients from one academic medical centre, women were 23% less likely than men to have their cholesterol managed (Persell *et al.*, 2005). Hendrix *et al.* (2005) analysed the care of 72 508 people with hypertension who were treated in the USA. More men than women received definitive diagnoses of angina, while more women than men were diagnosed with vague chest pain. Also, women received fewer cardiovascular medications than men. Use of a low-dose aspirin regimen reduces the risk of heart attack and stroke, and reduces heart disease deaths. Opotowsky *et al.* (2007) examined data on 1869 men and women aged 40 or older who reported heart disease prior to a heart attack. After adjusting for demographic, socioeconomic, and clinical characteristics, 62% of women reported regular aspirin use, compared with 76% of men.

In a study of more than 9000 Michigan Medicare patients, it was found that women undergoing coronary artery bypass graft surgery were 3.4 times as likely as men to have received blood transfusions (Rogers *et al.*, 2006). Patients who received a transfusion were more than three times as likely to develop an infection as those who did not, and they were 5.6 times as likely to die within 100 days after surgery. It was assumed that the presence of foreign leucocytes in donor blood may have suppressed the immune system of the recipients, thus increasing the risk of postoperative infection.

WORK TASKS

In countries where women have a paid job almost as often as men, the labour market tends to be gender segregated in several aspects. First, women more often than men have jobs in the public service sector, such as in hospitals and schools, whereas men are more often employed in the private sector. Second, women are more often found in low-status jobs with less influence and control over the pace and content of their work, which according to the Demand–Control theory contributes to stress and health problems. In addition, women workers are concentrated in a relatively limited number of jobs (health care workers, teachers, office work, shop assistants) compared with men, who are employed in a wider range of different jobs.

The 10 most prevalent occupations for employed women in the USA in 2008 (US Department of Labor, 2008) were:

1. Secretaries and administrative assistants.
2. Registered nurses.
3. Elementary and middle school teachers.
4. Cashiers.
5. Retail salespersons.
6. Nursing, psychiatric and home health aides.
7. First-line supervisors/managers of retail sales workers.
8. Waiters and waitresses.
9. Receptionists and information clerks.
10. Bookkeeping, accounting, and auditing clerks.

The 10 most common occupations for men were:

1. Drivers/sales workers and truck drivers.
2. Managers.
3. First-line supervisors/managers of retail sales workers.
4. Labourers and freight, stock, and material movers.
5. Construction labourers.
6. Retail salespersons.
7. Janitors and building cleaners.
8. Carpenters.
9. Sales representatives, wholesale and manufacturing.
10. Cooks.

Even when men and women are holding the same position, for example as a physician, men and women tend to do different things and choose different specialities. Women doctors more often than men work with children, geriatric and psychiatric patients, and chronically ill patients, and men more often work as general practitioners, surgeons and cardiologists. This is likely to influence work-related stress differently in women and men. Women doctors more often work in areas that are emotionally taxing. For example, long-term treatment of a geriatric or psychiatric patient creates a personal relationship and prognosis is often poor. In contrast male doctors have relatively short contact with their patients and the prognosis of their patients is more often good. This contributes to the more emotional engagement in patients by female doctors, which makes it more difficult to relax from work even during breaks and after work. In keeping with this, women doctors often report high levels of stress, and several studies report higher rates of suicide among female doctors compared with their male colleagues and the general population (Schernhammer & Colditz, 2004).

Frankenhaeuser *et al.* (1989) and Lundberg and Frankenhaeuser (1999) compared stress levels in male and female managers matched for age, education and occupational position, and found that women's stress levels remained elevated after work whereas men rapidly returned to their rest levels by the end of the workday (Fig. 10.1). Stress levels at work and at home in women, but not in men, have been found to be highly correlated (Lundberg, 1996). Men's physiological stress responses at work seem to be mainly related to their perceived

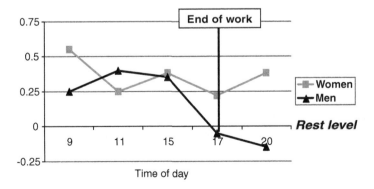

Fig. 10.1   Increase in noradrenaline (pmol/min/kg) during and after work among female and male managers. Reprinted from Lundberg & Frankenhaeuser (1999) with permission.

stress and work demands, whereas women's stress responses appear to reflect the interaction between stress at work and stress off work. A possible explanation is that women at work are stressed not only by their ongoing work tasks, but also by unpaid work responsibilities waiting at home, such as the need to decide what to eat for dinner, how to find time for food shopping, when and how to pick up children from day care or school, etc. Compared with male workers women also seem to think more about work and to ruminate about stressful events in their job (conflicts, unfinished tasks, deadlines, etc.) when they come home in the evening, and also seem to prepare themselves more carefully for meetings and events the following day. In interviews female managers often claim that they have to be more qualified and better prepared than their male colleagues to compete for the same positions. Klumb *et al.* (2006) examined paid and unpaid work in 52 dual-earner couples, and found that more paid work by the individual and his/her spouse tended to be associated with increased cortisol levels. In manual jobs, women are more often performing repetitive tasks, for example data entry, assembly work in the electronics industry, and work in the textile industry (sewing, making clothes), jobs which are known to increase stress levels and which are associated with slower unwinding after work and with a higher prevalence of MSD.

In conclusion, full-time employed women are often exposed to more stress at work and have fewer opportunities for rest and recovery off work compared with men. An alternative or additional possibility is that men and women differ in terms of vulnerability when exposed to work stress. As mentioned earlier (Krantz *et al.*, 2004), the relation between stress-induced muscular activity (EMG responses) and other physiological stress responses (blood pressure, heart rate) was much stronger in women than in men, which indicates a more generalised stress response in women than in men. Consistent sex differences in pain perception have also been demonstrated in humans (Hellström & Lundberg, 2000) and animals (Riley *et al.*, 1998; Sternberg, 1998), showing that females have a lower pain threshold than males. It has also been shown that gonadal hormones such as oestrogen are involved in pain regulation. For example, during pregnancy, pain thresholds are increased in animals (Gintzler, 1980), and pain ratings of women with chronic pain are lower during periods of high oestrogen levels (Hellström & Anderberg, 2003). Gender differences also exist in muscular mass and strength and in muscle fibre composition, which in some jobs may be relevant for the higher prevalence of muscular pain symptoms among women.

Gender differences in response to working shifts have been noted (Bara & Arber, 2009). On the basis of longitudinal data from the British Household Panel Survey 1995–2005, different types of shift work and night work were related to responses to the General Health Questionnaire. It was found that women's mental health was adversely affected by varied shift patterns whereas men's mental health was more negatively influenced by night work.

Tytherleigh *et al.* (2005) performed an analysis of data from the ASSET model of stress (Cartwright *et al.*, 2000), based on four main questionnaires with 12 subscales on perception of work, attitudes towards the organisation, health and biographical and demographical information, collected from 1974 full-time permanent university staff in 14 universities in the UK. It was found that men perceived low pay and insufficient benefits as greater sources of stress than did women. Participants between 36 and 45 years of age were most stressed, which corresponds to the peak in total workload found in full-time employed male and female white-collar workers between the ages of 30 and 40 years by Lundberg *et al.* (1994). It was concluded (Tytherleigh *et al.*, 2005), that 'the multivariate model suggests that gender differences in perceived stress of work relationships, work–life balance, overload, job security, control, resources and commitments, and job overall are better explained by

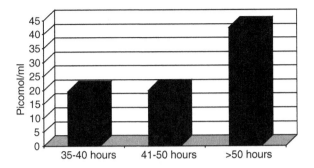

Fig. 10.2 Regular weekly paid workload and morning cortisol in women. Reprinted from Lundberg & Hellström (2002) with permission.

differences in age and/or job exposure factors of type of university, category of employee, salary, additional responsibilities and hours worked'. Gender differences in vulnerability were found to be of minor importance (Tytherleigh *et al.*, 2005). With regard to commitment, age and job factors were found to be more important than gender, and hours worked accounted for more variance in the model than any other factor on the scores for commitment. As expected, women reported higher levels of stress-related ill health than men, which was assumed to be due to gender differences in exposure to work stress. For example, women academics more often have to fulfil emotionally demanding roles involving teaching and interacting with students, whereas men are more likely to perform research and administrative duties.

Women working more than 60 hours per week reported lower levels of control, whereas men reported being more in control by doing so (Tytherleigh *et al.*, 2005). As mentioned in Chapter 7, women regularly working more than 50 hours per week have cortisol levels twice as high in the morning compared with women working fewer hours (Fig. 10.2; Lundberg & Hellström, 2000). These findings can be related to results from the previous study (Alfredsson *et al.*, 1985) which showed that women working more than 10 hours extra every week (i.e. more than 50 hours per week) had significantly increased risk of myocardial infarction during the coming year compared with women's normal risk. Women's traditionally greater responsibility for home and children means that their opportunities for rest and recovery are very much restricted during periods with long working hours. For example, Rissler (1977) measured stress hormone levels (adrenaline and noradrenaline) in women office workers during a period of quantitative overload (up to 15 hours extra per week). The extra hours were worked during the weekend but adrenaline levels showed a significant increase in the evening at home in the middle of the week, which followed the number of extra hours worked with a delay of about a week. Lundberg and Palm (1989) compared the relation between number of overtime hours at work during a week and adrenaline levels during the following weekend in mothers and fathers with preschool children, and found a significant positive association in mothers but not in fathers in the same families. This means that women's, but not men's, amount of overtime in their paid job is reflected in their stress hormone levels in the weekend. A likely explanation for this gender difference is that the extra hours at work reduced the time for shopping, cleaning, doing the washing and other household chores during the week and forced the mothers (but not necessarily the fathers) to perform more unpaid work at weekends. More on gender differences in unpaid work is presented in the next section.

UNPAID WORK AND TOTAL WORKLOAD

In addition to paid work, a large amount of valued work tasks and services are also carried out as unpaid work. Examples are household duties, childcare, care of sick and elderly relatives and voluntary work in various organisations (Kahn, 1991). Studies in Europe and other parts of the world consistently show that women spend more time in unpaid work than do men. Examples are shopping for food and clothes, cooking, cleaning, doing the washing, sewing, mending, ironing, remembering birthdays and other celebrations, buying presents, taking care of small children, changing nappies, helping children with school work, etc. In addition to performing the actual tasks, women more often carry the main responsibility for these tasks, for example they have to plan ahead and remind the rest of the family about when it is time for major cleaning, changing of bed linen or curtains, watering flowers, preparing for birthdays, etc., even if they do not have to perform the actual tasks themselves. Exceptions are three areas for which men often take the main responsibility. These areas are repair and maintenance of the house/flat, the car and managing finances.

In 1990 and 2001 Swedish studies (Lundberg *et al.*, 1994; Berntsson *et al.*, 2005) were performed to examine paid and unpaid workload in full-time employed and highly educated women and men, matched for age, occupation and number of children. Groups of about 1000 men and 1000 women were selected, consisting of an equal number of male and female physicians, psychologists, administrators, chemists and other academic groups. The participants were requested by means of questionnaires to estimate the number of hours they spent in their paid job, and in different activities in the household and in childcare and other unpaid tasks during a normal week. It was found that women had a higher weekly total workload of about five hours up to the age of 50, above which the gender differences disappeared, and that workload increased with the number of children in the family (Lundberg *et al.*, 1994). In families without children, men and women spent about the same number of hours per week in unpaid work at home. However, in families with children, workload increased more among women. For example, in families with three children or more, the total workload for women was on average about 90 hours per week compared with about 72 hours for men. As both men and women had a full-time job of about 40 hours per week, this difference was due to unpaid work (household, children, etc.). When the study was replicated in 2001 (Berntsson *et al.*, 2005), 11 years later and with new groups selected in the same way, women were found to spend about one hour less per week and men one hour more in household work compared with the corresponding data from 1990. The gender difference of about five hours in total workload remained the same but the total weekly workload had increased about 10 hours for both women and men (Fig. 10.3). This increase in total workload between 1990 and 2001 was partly the result of a higher paid workload in both women and men, but also a consequence of spending more time caring for their children and for sick and elderly relatives and on voluntary work. With regard to responsibilities for household chores and child care, no change had occurred between 1990 and 2001.

This means that even when women and men have a full-time job in the same position and choose to combine their occupational career with family responsibilities, women often have a much greater total workload and more responsibility for unpaid work. One explanation for the pronounced difference in unpaid work between the matched groups of men and women just discussed (Lundberg *et al.*, 1994) with three children or more is that a full-time working man in a high-status job, for example a male physician, often has a part-time working wife taking care of home and children, whereas it is unusual for a full-time working female physician to have a part-time working husband doing the same thing. This is likely to cause

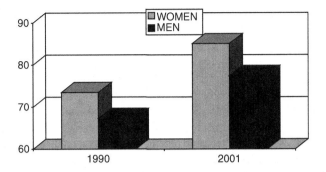

Fig. 10.3   Total weekly workload (number of hours in paid + unpaid work) of full-time-employed matched groups of male and female white-collar workers, 1990 (Lundberg *et al.*, 1994) and 2001 (Berntsson *et al.*, 2005).

more stress and role conflicts for full-time-employed women compared with men in families with children and to reduce the time for rest and recuperation.

Although the data above were based on highly educated Swedish women and men, studies from other countries show a similar pattern (Cooper & Lewis, 1994; Gjerdingen *et al.*, 2000). As Sweden is considered to be quite highly developed in terms of gender equality, it was assumed that gender differences would be less pronounced than in other countries. As the costs of hiring domestic aid to reduce unpaid work at home have been too high to be an option for most Swedish families, household chores have almost always been performed by family members as unpaid work at home. However, a recently introduced possibility for tax deduction of costs for domestic help may change this situation.

Women's participation in the paid workforce has increased in most countries in recent decades, for example in the EU from 51% in 1997 to 57% in 2006. In the 25 EU countries in 2003, the employment rate was 71% for men and 55% for women. In the USA about 60% of women aged 16 years and over were active within the labour force in 2008, about 25% of them on a part-time basis. According to *The Economist* (2005), women account for 46.5% of the USA's workforce but are less than 8% of its top managers. In countries with limited or no access to affordable childcare (e.g. Germany and the UK), women often have to make a choice between an occupational career and having family and children.

Fielden and Cooper (2002) found that women in senior status positions are at great risk of stress-related illness owing to feelings of isolation and loneliness. Women who occupy full-time jobs in demanding professional roles are exposed to multiple conflicts between demands from work and family. A man in a similar position is allowed to neglect domestic work and family in favour of his career demands, whereas a female top manager is also expected to fulfil her maternal role and be a good mother, spend time with and be committed to her children, run her home properly, dress nicely and look pretty. She is often also expected to be a good wife and support her husband's career achievements.

Simon (1995) examined gender differences in 40 employed married parents in the USA with regard to mental health associated with combining spouse, parent and worker roles. It was concluded that work and family roles have different meanings for males and females, which could explain why women's mental health benefits less from multiple roles compared with men's mental health. Women believed that their role as mother and wife involved more than economic support and that their employment was competing with their obligations to meet family needs. In contrast, men felt that their employment was the most important contribution to their role as father and husband. Of the women 70% indicated that they often felt inadequate as mothers and wives, whereas 90% of the men considered themselves to be successful fathers and husbands. More women than men felt that combining work and parenthood had adverse consequences for their marriage, and they assumed a greater responsibility for marital problems. These results reflect a traditional gender role perspective, with men's major role being a breadwinner and women being mainly responsible for home and family even when both parents are in gainful employment. A woman's work role is assumed not to interfere with her other roles. This view expressed by employed parents in the USA in 1995 may have changed to some extent and can be expected to differ from that in countries where women's participation in the workforce started much earlier and is now of the same magnitude as that for men. However, as illustrated above with data from Sweden, these gender roles are still very widespread even in countries with 'gender equality' policies and more employed women. Feelings of guilt for neglecting children, home and family matters are still more pronounced among women than among men (Elvin-Novak, 1999).

CHILDREN, WOMEN AND STRESS

Children seem to play an important role in employed women's stress levels. Luecken *et al.* (1997) examined the effects of having children at home in 109 employed women and found that women with children reported higher levels of home strain and excreted significantly more cortisol than women without children at home. Similarly, Lundberg and Frankenhaeuser (1999) measured catecholamine levels during and after work in matched groups of 30 male and 30 female managers, finding that women with children at home had higher noradrenaline levels after work than women without children and than men, regardless of whether the men had children or not. In conclusion, full-time-employed women with children have fewer opportunities for rest and restitution off work compared with men and women without children at home.

Women's greater involvement in childcare compared with men's does not have to be stressful in itself. On the contrary, close interaction with children is likely to be rewarding and to contribute to well-being, satisfaction and meaningfulness in life. Nevertheless, inability to relax, sleep and recuperate leads to health risks in the long term.

By choosing to work part-time, the total workload can be reduced, but this causes negative consequences for future occupational career opportunities, and has both short- and long-term economic consequences including pension benefits after retirement. Often women, but very seldom men, decide to reduce their own paid work when they have small children. Since many couples separate before retirement, this means that women who divorce may have to reduce their economic standard considerably even after retirement, whereas their former husband may enjoy a higher income and pension as he has been able to work full-time and has made a successful career thanks to his former wife taking care of home and children.

11   Preventive Strategies

OCCUPATIONAL HAZARDS

In a large part of the world, physical hazards at work are still the most important reasons for morbidity and mortality among workers. Examples are exposure to poisonous and dangerous chemicals, pollution, and physical risks at work causing accidents. The most important first step to improve health is to reduce or eliminate such risks. In Europe and North America, physical occupational health risks are to a large extent controlled by rules and regulations. In some countries, important psychosocial risk factors have been identified and recommendations have been made on how to create a more healthy work situation (Health and Safety Executive, HSE, 2009). Examples of psychosocial work conditions that should be avoided in order to improve health are repetitive, monotonous and machine-paced work tasks, static load, marginalisation and social isolation. Measures to create a more healthy work situation could be job rotation and other forms of variation, education and 'empowerment'. 'Empowerment' or 'engagement' includes, among other things, improved opportunities, autonomy, encouragement, and development of skills.

HEALTH PROMOTION

In Chapter 9 various forms of health promotion were described that represent empirical workplace interventions that aim not only to reduce health risks, but also to contribute to a more healthy work situation and feelings of well-being. Some of these interventions have been linked to biological parameters, and to new research on positive psychology and the role of restorative environments, recuperation and sleep for the stimulation of anabolic bodily processes. Investments to improve work conditions are sometimes treated as 'unnecessary' costs, which are considered to reduce the company's competitiveness and profit. Some companies therefore choose to move manufacturing to countries with a less regulated labour market in terms of working hours, employment contracts and payment, such as China, India and Mexico, where in addition the physical and psychosocial work conditions are often worse. For workers in these countries, however, just having a paid job is usually considered to outweigh the risks associated with the work situation, and therefore they are unlikely to complain.

The Science of Occupational Health: Stress, Psychobiology and the New World of Work, first edition
By Ulf Lundberg and Cary L. Cooper. Published 2011 by Blackwell Publishing Ltd
© 2011 Ulf Lundberg and Cary L. Cooper

OCCUPATIONAL CONDITIONS IN EUROPE

Occupational conditions, rules and legislation vary to some extent within the EU. With a more liberal and global economy and a free market within the EU, workers, companies and capital can move between countries. This creates more competition and sometimes irritation and frustration, when workers from a poorer country compete for jobs with those in an affluent country who earn much higher pay. Whereas companies have become global and can move capital and goods between countries, the labour unions are mainly national, although some international collaboration occasionally occurs. Multinational companies and the deregulation of the labour market have reduced the power of the unions. This has decreased interest in being a union member. In Sweden, for instance, where 82% of all workers were union members ten years ago, the corresponding figure today is 72%. All major unions except the academic trade union (SACO) have lost members during this period.

The economic crisis starting in 2008 affected countries in the EU differently. The countries that were most influenced by the crisis were Spain, Ireland and the Baltic countries, with the unemployment rate doubling or in case of the Baltic countries nearly trebling. In March 2009 the unemployment rate in Spain was 17.4%, in Ireland 10.6% and in Latvia 16.1%. By comparison, in March 2009 the average unemployment rate was 8.9% in the 27 EU countries, 9.5% in Europe as a whole and 8.6% in the USA. Following a period of rapid economic growth in the Baltic countries after independence from the former Soviet Union, the recession caused a banking crisis. Foreign capital has been invested in increasing amounts during the last two decades but has not been balanced with growth in exports. This has caused enormous debts to foreign banks, a reduced gross national product (GNP), big deficits in national budgets and a very high unemployment rate. In order to obtain additional economic support and create a balanced budget, workers' pay has been reduced considerably and taxes have increased. A similar severe financial crisis, with a foreign debt 10 times the annual national gross domestic product, hit Iceland and forced the prime minister to resign. Since then Greece has had severe economic problems, with considerable consequences for the EU and the euro. In these situations, the general interest in and efforts to reduce psychosocial stress at work and improve well-being among employees are not very strong. However, the allostatic load on employees who remain in work, as well as on those who have lost their jobs, is presently very high, and is likely to be reflected in increasing stress-related disorders within the next few years. As mentioned earlier, there is already a high prevalence of CVD among workers in the Baltic states compared with western Europe, and this has been associated with the psychosocial stress to which populations have been exposed during recent decades as a result of extensive political, economic and social changes (Kristenson, 1998).

HEALTHY WORK

A work situation not leading to exhaustion and distress but instead contributing to stimulation, interest, learning, pleasure, well-being and health is of course always preferable for many reasons. One reason is that even a very demanding but stimulating work situation is likely to be followed by mental unwinding and a rapid return to physiological baseline levels after work, which, according to Allostatic Load Theory (McEwen, 1998), is necessary for long-term health. In contrast, a stressful work situation characterised by distress and job dissatisfaction contributes to keep stress levels elevated after work, and is likely to cause sleep problems and hence to induce allostatic overload. In addition, although both negative and positive work stress are associated with elevated adrenaline and noradrenaline levels, the HPA axis and cortisol secretion (described in Chapter 6 and related to a number of serious mental and physical disorders) seem to be more affected by negative and chronic work stress.

Important components of a healthy job are adequate levels of autonomy, responsibility, variation and complexity, meaningfulness of work tasks, learning opportunities, positive feedback, managerial support and a supportive culture (Cooper *et al.*, 2001). To be motivated, and to have a goal and a plan of how to reach this goal, create a good platform for carrying out the job and ultimate success in it. This sequence of events could be more or less regulated. The job of an assembly worker, a cashier or a ticket officer is very much regulated, and there are limited opportunities for learning. In less regulated jobs, such as the job of an architect, a journalist, a manager or a researcher, work continuously creates new challenges that need to be tackled, and which, like the physical training of an athlete, lead to successive learning of new things. Combined with communication and collaboration with others, and development of new methods and systems, this can create a higher level of competence and success. This does not mean that all work tasks have to be complex and creative. It is usually not possible to be 100% creative and focused all the time. A combination of work tasks with differing degrees of complexity is likely to be more optimal from a healthy work perspective. For example, a mentally demanding work situation, such as complex problem solving, emotional work, being creative in new product development, and high-precision manual and mental work (such as neural and cardiac surgery), requires focused attention and emotional involvement and is associated with activation of important stress systems. Such demanding work tasks are often followed by tiredness and sometimes even by exhaustion. After such a work period, it is usually difficult to mobilise enough energy to continue to be creative, whereas simple routine tasks may be performed quite easily and even be perceived as relaxing.

Christensen (2008) has emphasised the difference between absence of negative work characteristics and positive experiences of job satisfaction and engagement, and has proposed a model for studying positive factors at work. The model is based on four factors:

1. Job resources (leadership practices and styles, innovative climate, job control).
2. Individual trait-like resources (efficacy beliefs, optimism).
3. Work-related experiences and attitudes (motivation, flow, work engagement).
4. Organisational and individual outcomes (retention, performance, well-being, long-term health).

SES AND HEALTH

Research on SES and health consistently demonstrates that a high status, a high income and a high level of education are health-promoting factors, but it has also been shown that great SES differences within a society are associated with reduced health. For example, the mean economic standard of living in terms of GNP in the USA ($38 000 per capita) is higher than in Sweden ($31 000 per capita), but the number of children dying before the age of one is twice as high in the USA (6.3 deaths/1000 live births) than in Sweden (3.2 deaths/1000 live births), and life expectancy is shorter in the USA (78.1 years) than in Sweden (80.9 years). This can be explained by the fact that a relatively large proportion (about 15%) of the American population is living below the level of poverty according to Federal norms, while at the same time some Americans are extremely rich. In Sweden, very few people are 'poor' and very few are extremely rich. According to the United Nations Children's Fund, UNICEF (2000), 22.4% of children in the USA live in poverty, compared with 2.6% in Sweden. This means that reduced variation in income may in some cases be more important for health than a general increase in mean income level, which is in line with the statistics reported by Wilkinson and Picket (2009). Access to qualified medical treatment and care is also likely to be an important factor. The USA has the highest health-care costs in the world, but a large part (at least 15%) of the population has no health insurance, which creates great individual differences with regard to access to advanced medical care among Americans. In several countries in Europe, most citizens are covered by a national medical insurance scheme and pay very little or nothing at all for medical treatment, medical care and medication. In Sweden, for instance, in 2010 the maximum annual costs paid for medical care and treatment by a single person were about $130 (SEK 900) and $250 (SEK 1800) for medication. A single visit to a general practitioner was about $20 (SEK 140) and $45 (SEK 320) to see a specialist. For children, all medical care and treatment were free of charge. Additional costs for treatment, care and medication were paid by the national health insurance financed via taxation.

WORK–LIFE BALANCE

The most important form of intervention to reduce stress-related disorders and improve well-being is not always to lower the mental and physical stress levels at work. It is possible to cope with a stressful job provided that that there are adequate opportunities for rest and recovery off work. It is also important for people to be able to combine work and other parts of life without work overload and conflicting demands. Such overload and conflict mean that conditions off work, such as relationships with partner, children and other relatives, and economic and psychosocial conditions at home, interact with stress from the work situation. Work conditions are known to spill over into non-work life, but conditions off work also influence the work situation. If this mutual negative influence between work and non-work life escalates over time, serious stress-related conditions, such as burnout syndromes, depression and chronic fatigue, may develop.

The difficulties of managing parenting and employment are particularly pronounced for dual-earner couples, and for single parents with small children. Despite policies to stimulate more men to become involved in caring and domestic work, work–life balance continues to be gender segregated with women retaining a much closer tie to family care and domestic responsibilities (Lewis et al., 2007). The European Foundation for the Improvement of Living and Working Conditions 2005 reports that on average 10% of men and women in the 25 EU countries have difficulties fulfilling their family and domestic responsibilities several times each week because of the amount of time they spend at work. Hochschild (1997) and Gatrell (2007) conclude that professionally and managerially employed fathers in the UK and USA are discouraged by employers from seeking part-time work. The masculine role is still associated with full-time breadwinning, willingness to sacrifice family in favour of work at the office and playing a minimal part in physical care of babies and the upbringing of children. A more equal division of childcare and domestic work between parents would thus be beneficial from a stress-reduction perspective.

The new forms of work with more flexibility could offer employees greater opportunities to influence their working conditions to suit individual needs, for example by reducing working hours, rearranging working times and working accordingly from home when it is possible. Although opportunities to work more 'flexibly' are theoretically open to both women and men, part-time work is seldom an option for men but is often used by women with small children. Men, on the other hand, may be expected to be flexible by working extra hours, sometimes with little or no extra pay. As concluded by Gatrell and Cooper (2008), 'the notion of 'flexibility' in relation to employed mothers and fathers may be interpreted by employers as both justification for placing working mothers on the "mummy track", and as an opportunity for intensifying fathers' workload'.

Even in the Nordic countries, where gender equality has been an issue for a long time, mothers are encouraged to work full time, and good childcare during working hours is readily available for most families at a low cost, gender differences in terms of work–life balance are pronounced. In Sweden, for instance, mothers and fathers are able to share equally the 390 days of paid parental leave following the birth of a new child. However, 60 days are reserved for each of the parents, and cannot be used by their spouses. A special bonus of about $15 (SEK 100) a day is given to couples who share the parents' days more equally. Although the amount of paternity leave is increasing slowly, fathers still use only 19% of the total number of days allowed, and 60% of men do not use any paternity leave at all during the first year of life of their child. In Norway, Brandth and Kvande (2002) studied the use of paternal leave and found that most male workers in non-management positions took advantage of the paid paternity leave, but only 47% of Norwegian fathers in senior management positions used paternity leave. Lammi-Taskula (2006, p. 95) concludes that 'policies promoting fathercare are more significant on the symbolic level of gender relations than on the level of actual division of labour between mothers and fathers'.

A poor work–life balance is associated with costs in terms of reduced well-being and increased stress levels (Swann & Cooper, 2005). According to a UK survey, 49% of parents expressed a desire to work fewer hours, and over 35% of working parents felt stressed (Worrall & Cooper, 1999). Pressures from combining parenting and employment also contributed to unhealthy lifestyles, including poor dietary habits, smoking, lack of exercise, increased alcohol intake, irritability and difficulties sleeping. In order to reduce sickness levels among working parents, especially in managerial and professional roles, a reduction in working hours for both men and women and a more gender-equal share of responsibility for childcare and household work would be necessary. Hindrances to this development are traditional gender role patterns in terms of 'male' and 'female' work and economic conditions. For example, because men usually earn more money, the costs of cutting down paid work hours are usually greater for men than for women. Therefore, women often have to pay the costs in terms of reduced income from a short- as well as a long-term perspective, and reduced career opportunities.

WHAT CAN WE DO TO REDUCE STRESS?

Some general recommendations

Individual level

- What makes you feel good: singing, music, dance, hobbies, nature? Try to give priority to things that are important in your life.
- Keep close social and emotional relationships with family and friends.
- Make the total workload more gender equal.
- Improve your lifestyle with regard to dietary habits, smoking, alcohol, exercise and sleep.
- Practise stress management and relaxation training when possible.

Organisational level

- Give the ability to influence pace and content of work, and have flexible work schedules.
- Ensure variation and development at work.
- Offer help and support when needed.
- Give appreciation and adequate reward for effort.

Societal level

- Social and economic justice.
- A reasonable work–life balance.

COMMENTS ON PREVENTIVE STRATEGIES

In conclusion, preventative strategies to promote occupational health should preferably be made on an organisational and societal level to affect as many people as possible, but influencing individual behaviour towards a more healthy lifestyle is also important. In Chapter 9, examples of organisational and individual interventions to reduce mental and physical health risks at work and to reduce stress and promote rest, recovery and restorative behaviour were presented. With regard to more large-scale societal interventions, political action to reduce socioeconomic differences, to provide affordable high-quality health care to all citizens and to create opportunities for a reasonable work–life balance, for example by offering affordable childcare, economic incentives for families with children to share paid and unpaid work more equally, and flexible working arrangements, seem to be of particular importance.

12 The Future Workplace from a Stress–Health Perspective

A CHANGING WORLD

Occupational stress research has consistently shown that 'work' can be positive and does not have to cause health problems. On the contrary, a paid job usually contributes to well-being and health ('the spice of life'), but under certain conditions, work can also be an important source of stress and involve exposure to physical and mental hazards ('a kiss of death'). The relationships between work and health are complex, and include interactions between individual characteristics, biological and behavioural factors, organisational and work-related factors as well as economic and political conditions in society. With an increasing rate of change in the workplace in terms of technology, communication, the economy and political policies, knowledge about these relationships becomes increasingly important for individual, occupational and public health professionals.

Modern communication technology, including the internet, emails, laptops and mobile phones, has had a dramatic effect on work conditions. This development has been combined with extensive economic changes, globalisation of economies, deregulation of the labour market (outsourcing, offshore manufacturing, lean production) and more flexible and insecure forms of employment (part-time work, temporary employment). The speed of development of communication and computerised technology is increasing. For example, ten years ago mobile phones were nothing but wireless telephones, but are now advanced computers with a high resolution colour display, access to the internet and email communication, an integrated video camera and GPS (Global Positioning System) technology and an MP3 player. Today, a large part of the population in the industrialised countries uses computers and mobile phones almost every day. In addition, new technology for automation, genetic manipulation and increased demands for more variation and development of new products have given rise to a constant need for repeated reorganisation at work and continuous adaptation to new working arrangements. In order to increase flexibility and adapt to changing conditions, many companies have replaced permanent employment by temporary and part-time employment by hiring personnel from employment services companies. Access to mobile and miniaturised electronic equipment has increased the employees' freedom and flexibility to work in a 'boundaryless' way, but having their staff

The Science of Occupational Health: Stress, Psychobiology and the New World of Work, first edition
By Ulf Lundberg and Cary L. Cooper. Published 2011 by Blackwell Publishing Ltd
© 2011 Ulf Lundberg and Cary L. Cooper

'on line' also means that the employers have gained more control over workers' performance and whereabouts.

The rate of change in occupational settings, and in society as a whole, is likely to continue to increase in an accelerated fashion. This will induce elevated demands on many individuals but also more opportunities and, hence, will create greater health differentials in society. For some individuals technological development, more flexible work conditions and a deregulated and global economy contribute to increasing resources, well-being and health, but for others this development may cause alienation, unemployment, reduced resources and impaired mental and physical health. In many cases, technological development has created new resources and advancements, such as increased medical resources to fight disease and improve health. As a result, the infant mortality rate has dropped by about 30% around the world during the past two decades, with the most dramatic improvements in countries in Asia and Africa. In 1900, world life expectancy was approximately 30 years, in 1985 it was about 62 years, and in 2007 about 64 years. However, there are still considerable health inequalities around the world, between as well as within nations, related to socioeconomic conditions (Marmot, 2008).

The accelerated rate of change in society is also inducing increasing demands on human adaptation resources. Although human beings, on balance, are very flexible, and are able to cope with stressful conditions and new demands, there are limits to adaptation and some individuals are more vulnerable than others, depending on biological factors as well as on earlier experiences, coping strategies and social and economic resources. Experiences early in life are important for these intra-individual differences.

WORK AND HEALTH

Worrying about economic problems and feeling insecure about the future are psychological conditions that affect individuals all the time. It is difficult to get rid of negative thoughts, and this kind of chronic stress will reduce opportunities for rest and recovery, which are necessary to balance periods of stress. The effects on sleep are of particular importance. Apprehension about future problems and demands reduces sleeping time and increases the number of awakenings. Zoccola et al. (2009) exposed 122 college undergraduates with different levels of trait rumination to an acute psychosocial stressor. Stressor-specific rumination was measured as the frequency of task-related thoughts 10 min after the stressor. Both trait and stressor-specific rumination predicted impaired sleep quality in terms of longer objective sleep onset latency, measured by actigraphs. Anticipation stress or rumination about stressful experiences reduced the most important form of sleep from a restitutional perspective, that is, deep or slow-wave sleep according to EEG measurements. Peiper and Brosschot (2005) and Brosschot et al. (2005) have emphasised the role of prolonged stress activation for stress-induced somatic disease, mediated through worry, rumination and anticipatory stress. Thus, ruminating about problems, and anticipatory worrying, may activate central processes in the body, which increase catabolism and reduce anabolism and restoration. From a long-term perspective, this imbalance between catabolic and anabolic bodily processes may cause dysregulation of physiological and endocrinological systems, and induce a spectrum of health problems.

Knowledge about occupational conditions contributing to the promotion of health, as well as conditions causing ill health, is important for treatment, intervention and prevention. It is also important to learn about the psychobiological mechanisms involved. This will help people to understand why symptoms appear and, hopefully, encourage them to take proper action before their condition gets worse. Stress influences the regulation of major bodily systems, but is not always reflected in clinical risk values in terms of blood pressure, lipids, glucose, etc. It seems that the dynamic regulation and the balance between different bodily systems are disturbed by chronic stress, which causes symptoms and disease. By learning more about how these negative effects can be identified and evaluated, for example in terms of high allostatic load and dysregulation of the HPA axis, biomarkers of stress can be used as reliable indicators of both a stressful work situation and an emerging health problem, and provide the means to evaluate interventions aimed at improving health in the work environment. By more 'objective' markers of unhealthy work conditions, such as physiological and psychological biomarkers of health, the motivation to change such conditions is usually higher than when only data on self-reported health and perceived stress levels are available.

Although the 'work–stress–health' relationship is complex, and the inter-individual variation in susceptibility to work-related stress is high and occupational conditions change rapidly over time, there is now a large body of scientific evidence on occupational health-damaging and health-promoting factors. Numerous studies have been published on occupational stress and health, as well as on the bodily responses to stress and the mechanisms linking stress responses to various health outcomes (Cooper *et al.*, 2009; Lundberg, 2009a,b). However, research comes from diverse areas, and knowledge obtained in different disciplines has usually not been combined and integrated. The aim of this book was to bring these fields together and lay the groundwork for more efficient means of health-promoting interventions in occupational settings, based on organisational research as well as biological facts. Although more research is always necessary, our general opinion is that there is already a vast literature representing the scientific evidence in this field. This knowledge needs to be combined and transformed into specific science-based actions in order to promote health in the future occupational environment.

Better nutrition, increased welfare, access to medical care, medical improvements and healthier lifestyles (improved dietary habits, reduced smoking, regular physical exercise) are some important factors contributing to increased longevity in all parts of the world. Improvements in the most disadvantaged parts of the world, where half of the population is dying before the age of 50, are most important for reducing infant mortality and increasing life expectancy. However, in the industrialised parts of the world also, people are expected to live longer in the future, but differences in health and longevity between social and occupational groups are considerable within these countries. For example, in the UK, life expectancy follows a gradient, and in the highest SES group (social class I) is 7.4 years longer than in the lowest (social class V). Europeans in general are expected to gain about 5 years in life expectancy by the year 2050. This will have profound demographic effects, with an increasing proportion of older people. In the 27 EU countries, the proportion of the population over the age of 65 will almost double in the next 40 years, which means that fewer working people will have to support a growing number of the elderly. At present there are about four people of working age for every one aged over 65, but in 2060 there will be only two for every one.

The strong association found in ten European countries (Lager & Bremberg, 2009) between young people's mental health problems and the proportion of young people excluded from the labour force is alarming in view of the high and increasing rate of unemployment in many countries and the trend of constantly increasing mental health problems among young people (girls in particular) in recent decades. According to WHO statistics (2006), the proportion of 15-year-old girls experiencing sadness, nervousness, irritation and sleeping problems more than once a week in 1985 was about 20%. In 2005 this figure had increased to over 40%. For boys the corresponding increase was from about 10% to 20%. In Sweden reports of anxiety and worrying among women aged 16–24 years increased from 10% in 1989 to 30% in 2005 (Statistics Sweden, 2006).

A likely explanation for this trend is that young people today learn from mass media, the internet and various authorities about the opportunities available to them to get an appropriate education, followed by a stimulating well-paid job and an exciting occupational career. Schoolchildren and students are informed about all possible lines of education, national as well as international, that are available, and they get the impression that it is all up to themselves, their ambitions and their efforts to be successful in their education and on the labour market. However, when they face the realities, things are different. There is usually very strong competition for the most attractive educational options, and not all young people have the mental, social or economic resources to compete for and be accepted for the courses. For those who succeed and are accepted, not everyone has the capacity to complete the course and pass the examinations. Stress levels are known to be high and mental health problems are common among students because of high demands, examination pressures, and uncertainty about future prospects on the labour market because of economic conditions at the time. This creates a dissociation between expectations induced by the information young people receive and the real world, which is likely to cause frustration and disappointment and induce mental distress. Some young people do not even try to get a formal education or training, because they feel at an early stage that they do not have the mental or physical capacity, and lack influence and economic and social resources to compete for and complete an education. As mentioned earlier, only a small part of the present labour market is open for people without formal training and education. For many young individuals this means a situation characterised by hopelessness, according to the CATS model ('Whatever I do, I will fail'). These young people may never get a permanent job and are likely to be unemployed for large parts of their adult life, which creates feelings of meaninglessness in life and causes distress, anxiety, worry, depression, economic problems and increased risk of physical symptoms, antisocial behaviour and drug abuse. Furthermore, young people striving and competing for attractive educational opportunities without succeeding are likely to respond with disappointment, distress and feelings of helplessness.

STRESS, WELL-BEING AND PRODUCTIVITY

There is growing evidence to suggest that reduced well-being and the resulting ill-health have a significant impact on organisational productivity and profitability. For example, Kessler and Frank (1997) estimated that, in terms of depression, monthly productivity losses of approximately $200 to $400 were experienced by each worker. Similarly, Greenberg *et al.* (1993) estimate that lost productivity due to depression costs American corporations $12.1 billion in 1990 alone.

Beyond these estimates, there are few empirical studies of the relationship between work stressors, well-being and productivity that have large samples and robust measures. Such studies are important since they would provide further compelling impetus to employers to ensure that appropriate working conditions are maintained, and would add to management's understanding of the role of stress in organisations.

Johnson (2009) did the first large-scale study of this, examining the relationship between stress and productivity in workers employed in a range of occupations. To achieve this, they used ASSET (Faragher *et al.*, 2004) which incorporates individual work stressors, stress outcomes (employee health) and commitment. By correlating ASSET's dimensions to self-report productivity, they examined the linkages between stress-related factors and productivity. ASSET was devised as a short stress-evaluation tool that can be completed quickly and easily by all employees within an organisation. It encompasses three areas related to workplace stress, including employee perceptions of the job (source of workplace stress and job pressure), commitment (both from and to the organisation) and employee health (physical health and psychological well-being). Productivity was measured through a self-report measure (Faragher *et al.*, 2004) and has been used in numerous empirical studies and found to have predictive validity in research into bullying at work (Einarsen *et al.*, 2003).

Data was collected from 16 001 employees across 15 different organisations in the UK. Respondents worked in a range of professional, administrative and manual occupations, 62% were female, 85% worked full-time, and ages ranged from 18 to over 60 years. Multivariate and univariate outliers and cases with more than 20% missing data were removed from the dataset. Remaining missing values were substituted with the mean response. A two-stage procedure was implemented with 80% of the sample used for model development and 20% used in cross-validation. The model development sample was submitted to a stepwise regression analysis. Three factors significantly predict approximately 23% of the variance in employee productivity. Specifically, the model suggests that higher employee productivity is associated with:

1. Better psychological well-being.
2. Higher perceived commitment from the organisation.
3. Greater access to resources and information.

Inspection of the cross-validation sample revealed a significant correlation between predicted and actual scores on the productivity measure, thereby providing support for the regression model.

Improvement of well-being in the workforce has been shown to be cost-effective. Improved health and performance seem to be strongly related to work engagement. For example, according to recent research on well-being in the UK on workplace health and well-being (Robertson Cooper, 2008), raising the levels of well-being by just 7% will potentially lead to savings of £12 billion per year in the UK. Kent County Police, who used ASSET to measure well-being, found that in just two years initiatives to increase well-being and health in the organisation led to a 25% reduction in sickness absence, which would equate to a saving of nearly £1.5 million per annum. Thus, despite difficulties in convincing organisations of investments for improving well-being of the workforce, there is considerable evidence of the economic and health benefits of such investments. By the use of biomarkers of stress and well-being, we are able to evaluate repeatedly over time the outcome of such interventions before hard evidence of health effects such as disease, sickness absence, labour turnover, reduced quality of work and conflict become visible. These measures also mean that improvements in interventions can be made at an early phase, in cases where the results according to the biomarkers are not satisfactory.

In conclusion, the results show a number of interesting relationships. First, the strongest predictor of productivity is psychological well-being. In accordance with existing research on burnout, a second influential factor is commitment from the organisation to the employee. Previous studies have shown a negative relationship between emotional exhaustion (a component of burnout) and productivity. Negative mental well-being is generally accepted as an antecedent of burnout. Therefore, the finding that well-being impinges negatively on productivity suggests that decrements to performance are likely to be evident earlier in the stress/burnout experience.

This investigation into the precursors of decreased productivity extends prior research through the inclusion of work stressors in the analysis. However, with the exception of 'resources and communication', no stressors were found to have a direct influence on productivity rates. It was proposed that resources have a direct impact on productivity as a result of the inability to perform effectively without the 'tools of the job' rather than through a stressor–stress pathway. The implication, therefore, is that individual work stressors have only an indirect effect on productivity through their impact on mental well-being.

DEMOGRAPHIC CHANGES IN EUROPE AND JAPAN

The future challenges in Europe and some other countries such as Japan from an ageing workforce and an increasing proportion of retired people is putting pressure on politicians to encourage a greater number of citizens to enter and remain in the workforce. Women are of particular interest in this context. Although female employment in large parts of the world has grown in recent years, there is still great potential for more women to enter the labour market. In order to achieve a higher employment rate among women, affordable and high-quality childcare, based on children's needs for social and personal development rather than economic motives, is a key factor. In the Nordic countries, where high-quality child daycare is already available at a low cost, women's employment rate is about the same as that of men, although more women than men work part-time when they have small children at home. We also need to increase the proportion of retired people active in the workforce by encouraging and helping elderly people to remain in employment for longer if they so choose. This can be done by adapting work practices, ergonomic design and health and safety programmes to take account of older people's needs, abilities and capacities, and to provide more support and assistance where and when required. More flexible forms of employment, such as part-time work and temporary work, are likely to fit older workers' needs better than those of younger workers, for whom stable work and economic conditions are necessary for independence and security.

Migrant workers are usually young people and may contribute to support the growing ageing population in Europe, both financially as taxpayers, but also physically, by filling the increasing demand for a range of jobs. Eurostat expects that at least 40 million people will have migrated to the EU by 2050. Obstacles to migrants' participation in the workforce concern housing, education, language problems and in some cases discrimination. New migrants are usually forced, or select themselves as a result of relatives or fellow countrymen already living there, to live in housing areas characterised by a high concentration of social problems, unemployment and poverty, where their own possibilities of finding a job are small. Local authorities can facilitate integration by investments to improve housing and environmental conditions, reduce crime and antisocial behaviour, and make it easier to form enterprises and employ workers (e.g. via low-interest loans and less bureaucracy). Educational and language problems can be overcome by providing free or subsidised courses for new migrants in areas relevant for their chances to get a job. As the demand for care workers already exceeds the supply, helping migrants by education and training, combined with improvement of working conditions and raising pay levels in care services, are important means for meeting this demand and securing positive care for children and the elderly in the future.

The increase in mental health problems in the younger generation is alarming in view of the fact that these people represent the future workforce, the new political and industrial leaders and scientists, who among other things are expected to handle the demographic challenge and the global climate crisis. Their mental state will be very important for their chances of succeeding with these ventures. The strong association found between unemployment rate and mental health problems indicates that political actions to reduce unemployment among young people should receive high priority (Cooper *et al.*, 2001; Lager & Bremberg, 2009). Educational and job training programmes, economic incentives to employ young people and stimulation and support to form new enterprises could be part of such actions.

GLOBAL ISSUES

Occupational life in the industrialised countries and in a number of cities all over the world faces a number of important challenges in the near future. The European workforce is growing older, and a larger proportion of the population will leave the workforce for retirement, which means that the resources for medical and psychosocial care of a growing number of elderly people will increase. In addition, mental health problems in the younger generation, 15–25 years, are increasing rapidly. The trend towards more flexible organisations, more competition and a more global economy is likely to continue and perhaps even increase in pace. This will create more flexible forms of employment such as temporary and part-time work, more frequent reorganisations, changes in products and methods of production, and a higher labour turnover and need for constant re-education of employees. At the beginning of the previous century, work as a farmer was the dominating job in Europe and North America. During industrialisation, a growing number of workers successively moved from farming towards manufacturing work. Today, manufacturing work is declining in these countries, and 'knowledge-based' information technology is increasing rapidly. In the emerging economies, such as China and India, these changes are occurring much faster than they did in Europe and North America, and are strongly taxing the adaptive resources of the population. The range of health consequences of these changes are not yet known, but more stress-related disorders can be expected and the negative effects of lifestyle changes, such as increased cigarette smoking, more unhealthy diets and less physical activity, can already be seen. The environmental load from and in these countries, representing almost a third of the world's population, is increasing in terms of pollution and carbon dioxide emissions because of more transportation and private cars and rapidly growing industry in need of more energy and raw materials. Dealing with these problems will be a major global challenge, requiring enormous resources in terms of manpower, new technology and economic investment.

Regional and global problems, such as the demographic changes in Europe and the global warming of the Earth, are likely to have a strong impact on work conditions and health in future. In the developing countries the rapid pace of change of occupational, economic and social conditions will be of particular importance. These changes will tax individuals' adaptive resources, but are likely to be associated mainly with positive effects and an increase in the economic standard of living for large parts of the population. This contributes to increased quality of life, life expectancy and reduced infant mortality, but differences between social groups, regions and countries are expected to be great. For example, well educated people and more developed regions within countries are expected to benefit most from this development. Expected negative global health effects of the ongoing changes are more people being killed in traffic accidents, diseases related to increased pollution, unhealthy diets, overweight, cigarette smoking, and drug abuse, for example CVD, lung cancer, obstructive lung disease and Type 2 diabetes.

The financial crisis that started in 2008 is an example of how events in a few important economies rapidly affect all nations in the world. Intensive international trade, a global economy and efficient means of immediate communication of news all over the world have contributed to these effects. Psychological factors play an important role for economic development as expectations about future economic trends seem to have a greater influence on stock exchanges than the companies' actual business and financial state. Therefore, the ups and downs in the global economy are expected to become even more far-reaching, frequent and unpredictable in the future.

An economic recession is usually associated with reduced sickness absence, but not because people become healthier through the recession. More likely explanations are that people with reduced health tend to lose their jobs first and hence the remaining workers in general have better health. Another explanation is that people who remain in work avoid taking sick leave even when they are ill ('illness presenteeism'), because they are afraid of losing their job if they are absent from work. As a consequence, they strain their own personal resources close to or beyond their capacity (allostatic load) to stay at work. From earlier economic crises we have learned that the reduction in absenteeism, combined with elevated job strain, is likely to be followed by a backlash in terms of rapidly increasing long-term sickness absence. The most recent and future economic crises are likely to follow similar trends with first, increasing unemployment, elevated stress levels (allostatic load) and reduced sickness absence, followed by increased (long-term) health problems and absenteeism a few years later.

Another example of a phenomenon that is likely to have a dramatic influence on the future economy and health in all parts of the world is global warming of the Earth, or the 'greenhouse effect', considered to be mainly caused by the increased emission of carbon dioxide but which may be enhanced by the effects of a reduction of the sunshine reflected from Earth and increased methane release from the seafloor because of the reduced ice shelf. The increasing temperature on the Earth will have extensive effects on the climate and living conditions for all species in all parts of the world. The melting ice sheets in the South and the North Poles will cause an elevated sea level that will put large areas of land under water. It is also assumed that a warmer climate will cause more extreme weather, with severe droughts as well as severe floods, but uncertainty about the long-term consequences is high. The effects will differ between countries. Some countries in the North, such as those of northern Europe, are likely to experience mainly positive effects of a warmer climate, for example, in terms of better conditions for farming and milder winters without snow, which facilitate transportation and require less energy for heating. Possible negative effects expected from a warmer climate in the North are greater risks for the spread of tropical diseases and ecological changes with a new fauna and new plants, with unpredictable long-term consequences. An elevated sea level may cause serious problems for several countries in terms of health, economy, housing and migration, and large parts of some nations, such as the islands of Fiji and Bangladesh, will end up under sea level. The Maldives, the highest point of which is only 2.5 m above the present sea level, will vanish completely if the sea level increases as feared. By and large, the negative effects of global climate change will be most pronounced in the poor countries of Africa, South America and Asia.

With regard to the economic effects, global warming is expected to create a large number of new jobs necessary to reduce the negative effects and to try to stop the ongoing climate crisis. Important tasks are to reduce the use of and dependence on fossil fuels (oil, coal, natural gas) and increase investments in clean energy, developing new ideas and new technology necessary to reach these goals. The rapidly growing populations of India and many countries in Africa, combined with the economic growth in countries such as China, are expected to contribute strongly to the emission of carbon dioxide and global warming, even if the emission *per capita* is reduced. Feeding an increasing world population, expected to reach 9 billion people by 2050, is another major challenge. Since these are true global phenomena with serious consequences for all living organisms, the long-term effects on the labour market and people's health and well-being are likely to be immense.

On the positive side, we know from earlier experiences that improvements in occupational health can be obtained by interventions at different levels (individual, organisational, societal, global). Individuals suffering from stress-related disorders need help, and with knowledge about the cognitive and bodily factors involved, more efficient methods of treatment can be developed. Increased well-being among workers is associated with substantial savings from the reduced need for medical care, less absenteeism from work and increased productivity. The resources created this way are needed for future economic investments to cope with the demographic challenges and climate changes. We also know a lot more about how humans respond to elevated work stress, about the psychobiological mechanisms linking psychosocial stress to a number of stress-related disorders, and about the different ways of preventing and reducing cumulative stress load ('allostatic load'). Today in the industrialised countries the major health problems do not seem to be caused by high levels of mental and physical overload at work as such, but rather by insufficient rest, restitution and sleep due to unremitting stress and the constant pressure and stress of working life. Modern communication technologies contribute to this by making it possible and expected for workers to keep in constant contact with their employers and with customers and clients, and to follow the news media, entertainment, etc., 24 hours a day from almost any place and in any situation. Furthermore, the development towards a more rapid pace of change in society, and increasing demands on people to make their own choices and take greater responsibility for their lives, has increased individuals' influence and control. But this 'empowerment' also means that people have to be continuously active and to make repeated decisions of importance for their lives and economic situation. The transformation of public companies providing electricity, water, telephone, bus and train transportation, a mail service, investments for pension benefits, etc., as well as private enterprises competing with each other to offer their services, has created many options for the individual to influence his or her economic and social situation. However, in order to take advantage of these options, it is necessary to keep oneself continuously informed and up to date about prices and conditions in order to make the right choices, and new decisions have to be made repeatedly at short intervals as conditions and options change constantly. Although these options generally present a positive situation, they also constitute a mental load that taxes the individual's adaptive resources and reduces opportunities for rest and restitution – and individuals with fewer resources and education are more vulnerable than others.

References

Aboa-Éboulé, C., Brisson, C., Maunsell, E., *et al.* (2007) Job strain and risk of acute recurrent coronary heart disease events. *JAMA*, **298** (14), 1652–1660.

Adler, N.E., Marmot, M., McEwen, B. & Stewart, J. (Eds) (1999) Socioeconomic status and health in industrial nations: social, psychological and biological pathways. *Annals of the New York Academy of Science*, **896**, 1–503.

Alavinia, S.M., van den Berg, T.I.J., van Duivenbooden, C., Elders, L.A.M. & Burdorf, A. (2009) Impact of work-related factors, lifestyle, and work ability on sickness absence among Dutch construction workers. *Scandinavian Journal of Work Environment and Health*, **35** (5), 325–333.

Alehagen, S., Wijma, K., Lundberg, U., Melin, B. & Wijma, B. (2001) Catecholamine and cortisol reaction to child birth. *International Journal of Behavioral Medicine*, **8** (1), 50–65.

Alehagen, S., Wijma, B., Lundberg, U. & Wijma, K. (2005) Fear, pain and stress hormones during childbirth. *Journal of Psychosomatic Obstetrics & Gynecology*, **26** (3), 153–165.

Alfredsson, L., Spetz, C.L. & Theorell, T. (1985) Type of occupation and near-future hospitalization for myocardial infarction and some other diagnoses. *International Journal of Epidemiology*, **14** (3), 378–388.

Allvin, M., Aronsson, G., Hagström, T., Johansson, G. & Lundberg, U. (2011) *Boundaryless Work – Social Psychological Perspectives on the New Working Life.* Wiley-Blackwell, Oxford. (In press.)

Antoni, M.H., Cruess, D.G., Klimas, N., *et al.* (2002) Stress management and immune system reconstitution in symptomatic HIV-infected gay men over time: effects on transitional naive T cells (CD4$^+$ CD45RA$^+$CD29$^+$). *American Journal of Psychiatry*, **159**, 143–145.

Antoni, M.H., Lutgendorf, S.K., Cole, S.W., *et al.* (2006) Influence of bio-behavioural factors on tumour biology: pathways and mechanisms. *Nature Reviews Cancer*, **6** (3), 240–248.

Antonovsky, A. (1987) *Unraveling the Mystery of Health.* Jossey-Bass, San Francisco.

Artazcoz, L., Benach, J., Borell, C. & Cortès, I. (2005) Social inequalities in the impact of flexible employment on different domains of psychosocial health. *Journal of Epidemiology & Community Health*, **59** (9), 761–767.

Balkau, B., Deanfield, J.E., Després, J-P., *et al.* (2007) A study of waist circumference, cardiovascular disease, and diabetes mellitus in 168 000 primary care patients in 63 countries. *Circulation*, **116** (17), 1942–1951.

Bara, A-C. & Arber, S. (2009) Working shifts and mental health – findings from the British Household Panel Survey (1995–2005). *Scandinavian Journal of Work, Environment & Health*, **35** (5), 361–367.

Barefoot, J.C., Dahlstrom, W.G. & Williams R.B. (1983) Hostility, CHD incidence, and total mortality: A 25 year follow-up study of 255 physicians. *Psychosomatic Medicine*, **45** (1), 59–63.

Beckers, D.G.J. (2008) Overtime work and well-being: opening up the black box. PhD thesis, Radboud University Nijmegen, The Netherlands.

Beddington, J., Cooper, C.L., Field, J., *et al.* (2008) The mental wealth of nations. *Nature*, **455** (23), 1057–1060.

Belkic, K.L., Landsbergis, P.A., Schnall, P.L. & Baker, D. (2004) Is job strain a major source of cardiovascular disease risk? *Scandinavian Journal of Work, Environment, & Health*, **30** (2), 85–128.

Bendel, O., Bueters, T., von Euler, M., Ove Ogren, S., Sandin, J. & von Euler, G. (2005) Reappearance of hippocampal CA1 neurons after ischemia is associated with recovery of learning and memory. *Journal of Cerebral Blood Flow and Metabolism*, **25** (12), 1586–1595.

Bernard, B.P. (1997) Musculoskeletal disorders and workplace factors. A critical review of epidemiologic evidence for work-related musculoskeletal disorders of the neck, upper extremity, and low back. CDC, National Institute for Occupational Safety and Health, Atlanta, GA.

Berntsson, L., Krantz, G. & Lundberg, U. (2005) Total workload: the distribution of paid and unpaid work as related to age, occupational level and number of children among Swedish male and female white-collar workers. *Work & Stress*, **15**, 209–215.

Berridge, J., Cooper, C.L. & Highley, C. (1997) *Employee Assistance Programs*. John Wiley & Sons, Chichester.

Bigos, S.J., Battié, M.C., Spengler, D.M., *et al.* (1991) A prospective study of work perceptions and psychosocial factors affecting the report of back injury. *Spine*, **16** (1), 1–6.

Biron, C., Brun, J-P., Ivers, H. & Cooper, C.L. (2006) At work but ill: psychosocial work environment and well-being determinants of presenteeism propensity. *Journal of Public Mental Health*, **5** (4), 26–37.

Björntorp, P. & Rosmond, R. (2000) The metabolic syndrome – a neuroendocrine disorder? *British Journal of Nutrition*, **83** (Suppl. 1), S49–S57.

Black, D.S., Milam, J. & Sussman, S. (2009) Sitting-meditation interventions among youth: a review of treatment efficacy. *Pediatrics*, **124**, 532–541.

Blumenthal, J.A., Sherwood, A., Babyak, M.A., *et al.* (2005) Effects of exercise and stress management training on markers of cardiovascular risk in patients with ischemic heart disease: a randomized controlled trial. *JAMA*, **293** (13), 1626–1634.

Boos, N., Semmer, N.K., Elfering, A., *et al.* (2000) Natural history of individuals with asymptomatic disc abnormalities in magnetic resonance imaging: predictors of low back pain-related medical consultation and work incapacity. *Spine*, **25** (12), 1484–1492.

Bowles, D. & Cooper, C.L. (2009) *Employee Morale*. Palgrave Macmillan, London.

Brandth, B. & Kvande, E. (2002) Reflexive fathers: negotiating parental leave and working life. *Gender, Work and Organisation*, **9** (2), 187–203.

Britton, A. & Shipley, M.J. (2010) Bored to death? *International Journal of Epidemiology*, **39**, 370–371.

Broadbent, E., Petrie, K.J., Alley, P.G. & Booth, R.J. (2003) Psychological stress impairs early wound repair following surgery. *Psychosomatic Medicine*, **65** (5), 865–869.

Brosschot, J.F., Peiper, S. & Thayer, J.F. (2005) Expanding stress theory: prolonged activation and perseverative cognition. *Psychoneuroendocrinology*, **30** (10), 1043–1049.

Buckle, P.W. & Devereux, J.J. (2002) The nature of work-related neck and upper limb musculoskeletal disorders. *Applied Ergonomics*, **33** (3), 207–217.

Burke, R. & Cooper, C.L. (eds) (2007) *The Human Resources Revolution*. Elsevier, Oxford.

Burke, R. & Cooper, C.L. (eds) (2008) *Building More Effective Organizations: HR Management and Performance in Practice*. Cambridge University Press, Cambridge.

Burke, H.M., Fernald, L.C., Gertler, P.J. & Adler, N.E. (2005) Depressive symptoms are associated with blunted cortisol responses in very low-income women. *Psychosomatic Medicine*, **67**, 211–216.

Burton-Jones, A. (1999) *Knowledge Capitalism: Business, Work and Learning in the New Economy*. Oxford University Press, Oxford.

Canivet, C., Östergren, P.O., Choi, B., *et al.* (2008) Sleeping problems as a risk factor for subsequent musculoskeletal pain and the role of job strain: results from a one-year follow-up of the Malmö Shoulder Neck Study Cohort. *International Journal of Behavioural Medicine*, **15** (4), 254–262.

Carrico, A.W., Antoni, M.H. & Pereira, D.B., *et al.* (2005) Cognitive behavioral stress management effects on mood, social support, and a marker of antiviral immunity are maintained up to 1 year in HIV-infected gay men. *International Journal of Behavioral Medicine*, **12** (4), 218–226.

Cartwright, S. & Cooper, C.L. (2004) Personal interventions. In: *Handbook of Work Stress* (eds J. Barling & K. Kelloway). Erlbaum, New Jersey.

Cartwright, S. & Cooper, C.L. (eds) (2009) *The Oxford Handbook of Organizational Wellbeing*. Oxford University Press, Oxford.

Cartwright, S. & Whatmore, L. (2005) Stress and individual differences: implications for stress management. In: *A Research Companion to Organizational Health Psychology* (eds A. S. Antoniou & C. L. Cooper), pp. 163–173. Edward Elgar, Cheltenham.

Cartwright, S., Whatmore, L. & Cooper, C.L. (2000) Improving communications and health in a government department. In: *Healthy and Productive Work* (eds Murphy, L. & Cooper, C.L.). Taylor & Francis, London.

Caruso, C.C., Hitchcock, E.M., Dick, R.B., *et al.* (2004) Overtime and extended work shifts: recent findings on illnesses, injuries, and health behaviors. National Institute of Health and Human Services (NIOSH), Cincinnati (OH).

Castells, M. (1996–2000) *The Information Age: Economy, Society and Culture*, Vols I–III. Blackwell, Oxford.

Catley, D., Kaell, A.T., Kirschbaum, C. & Stone A.A. (2000) A naturalistic evaluation of cortisol secretion in persons with fibromyalgia and rheumatoid arthritis. *Arthritis Care & Research*, **13** (1), 51–61.

Chou, A., Wong, L., Weisman, S., *et al.* (2007) Commercial health plans show disparities between women and men in cardiovascular care. *Women's Health Issues*, **17**, 120–130 (AHRQ contract 290-040-018).

Christensen, M. (ed.) (2008) Positive factors at work. The First Report of the Nordic Project. Nordic Council of Ministers. TemaNord: 501.

Clow, A., Thorn, L., Evans, P. & Hucklebridge, F. (2004) The awakening cortisol response: methodological issues and significance. *Stress*, **7** (1), 29–37.

Cohen, A. (1993) Age and tenure in relation to organizational commitment: a meta-analysis. *Basic and Applied Social Psychology*, **14** (2), 143–159.

Cohen, S. (2005) The Pittsburgh Common Cold Studies: psychosocial predictors of susceptibility to respiratory infectious illness. *International Journal of Behavioral Medicine*, **12** (3), 123–131.

Cohen, S. & Wills, T.A. (1985) Stress, social support, and the buffering hypothesis. *Psychological Bulletin*, **98** (2), 310–357.

Cohen, S., Doyle, W.J. & Baum, A. (2006) Socioeconomic status is associated with stress hormones. *Psychosomatic Medicine*, **68** (3), 414–420.

Cohen, S., Doyle, W.J., Alper, C.M., Janicki-Deverts, D. & Turner, R.B. (2009) Sleep habits and susceptibility to the common cold. *Archives of Internal Medicine*, **169** (1), 62–67.

Cohen, S., Doyle, W.J., Turner, R.B., Alper, C.M. & Skoner, D.P. (2003) Emotional style and susceptibility to the common cold. *Psychosomatic Medicine*, **65** (4), 652–657.

Cohen, S., Frank, E., Doyle, W.J., Skoner, D.P., Rabin, B.S. & Gwaltney, J.M., Jr (1998) Types of stressors that increase susceptibility to the common cold in healthy adults. *Health Psychology*, **17** (3), 214–223.

Cohen, S., Hamrick, N., Rodriguez, M.S., Feldman, P.J., Rabin, B.S. & Manuch, S.B. (2002) Reactivity and vulnerability to stress-associated risk for upper respiratory illness. *Psychosomatic Medicine*, **64** (2), 302–310.

Commission on the Social Determinants of Health (2008) Closing the gap in a generation: health equity through action on the social determinants of health. World Health Organization, Geneva.

Conti, R., Angelis, J., Cooper, C., Faragher, B. & Gill, C. (2006) The effects of lean production on worker job stress. *International Journal of Operations & Production Management*, **26** (9), 1013–1038.

Cooper, C.L. (ed.) (2005) *Handbook of Stress, Medicine and Health* (2nd edition) CRC Press, Boca Raton, FL.

Cooper, C.L. & Dewe, P. (2008) Well-being, absenteeism, presenteeism: costs and challenges. *Occupational Medicine*, **58** (8), 522–524.

Cooper, C.L. & Finkelstein, S. (eds) (2009) *Advances in Mergers and Acquisitions*. Emerald Press, Bingley, Yorkshire.

Cooper, C.L. & Jackson, S. (eds) (1997) *Creating Tomorrow's Organizations*. John Wiley & Sons, Chichester.

Cooper, C.L. & Lewis, S. (1994) *The Workplace Revolution: Managing Today's Dual-Career Families*. Kogan Page, London.

Cooper, C.L. & Marshall, J. (1976) Occupational sources of stress: a review of the literature relating to coronary heart disease and mental ill health. *Journal of Occupational Psychology*, **49** (1), 11–28.

Cooper, C.L. & Sadri, G. (1991) The impact of stress counselling at work. *Journal of Social Behavior and Personality*, **6** (7), 411–423.

Cooper, C.L., Dewe, P. & O'Driscoll, M. (2001) *Organizational Stress: A Review and Critique of Theory, Research and Applications*. Sage Publications, London.

Cooper, C.L., Field, J., Goswani, U., Jenkins, R. & Sahakian, B. (eds) (2009) *Mental Capital and Wellbeing*. Wiley-Blackwell, Oxford.

Cortada, J.W. (ed.) (1998). *Rise of the Knowledge Worker*. Butterworth-Heinemann, Boston.

Crofford, L.J., Young, E.A., Engleberg, N.C., *et al.* (2004) Basal circadian and pulsatile ACTH and cortisol secretion in patients with fibromyalgia and/or chronic fatigue syndrome. *Brain Behaviour & Immunity*, **18** (4), 314–325.

Desmeules, J.A., Cedraschi, C., Rapiti, E., *et al.* (2003) Neurophysiologic evidence for a central sensitization in patients with fibromyalgia. *Arthritis & Rheumatism*, **48** (5), 1420–1429.

Devereux, J., Rydstedt, L., Kelly, V., Weston, P. & Buckle, P. (2004) The role of work stress and psychological factors in the development of musculoskeletal disorders. Research Report 273. Robens Centre for Health Ergonomics for the Health and Safety Executive.

Dewe, P., O'Driscoll, M. & Cooper, C.L. (2010) *Coping with Workplace Stress*. Wiley-Blackwell, Oxford.

Dhabhar, F.S. & McEwen, B.S. (1997) Acute stress enhances while chronic stress suppresses cell-mediated immunity *in vivo*: a potential role for leukocyte trafficking. *Brain, Behavior and Immunology*, **11** (4), 286–306.

Dias-Ferreira, E., Sousa, J.C., Melo, I., *et al.* (2009) Chronic stress causes frontostriatal reorganization and affects decision-making. *Science*, **325** (5940), 621–625.

Dynesen, A.W., Haraldsdóttir, J., Holm, L. & Astrup, A. (2003) Sociodemographic differences in dietary habits described by food frequency questions – results from Denmark. *European Journal of Clinical Nutrition*, **57** (12), 1586–1597.

Einarsen, S., Hoel, H., Zapf, D. & Cooper, C.L. (2003) *Bullying and Emotional Abuse in the Workplace*. Taylor & Francis, London.

Ekstedt, M., Åkerstedt, T. & Söderström, M. (2004) Microarousals during sleep are associated with increased levels of lipids, cortisol, and blood pressure. *Psychosomatic Medicine*, **66** (6), 925–931.

Elfering, A., Gregner, S., Semmer, N.K. & Gerber, H. (2002) Time control, catecholamines and back pain among young nurses. *Scandinavian Journal of Work Environment & Health*, **28** (6), 386–393.

Elfering, A., Semmer, N.K., Birkhofer, D., Zanetti, M., Holder, J. & Boos, N. (2002) Risk factors for lumbar disc degeneration. A 5-year prospective MRI study of asymptotic individuals. *Spine*, **27**, 125–134.

Elfering, A., Semmer, N.K., Schade, V., Grund, S. & Boos, N. (2002) Supportive colleague, unsupportive supervisor: the role of provider-specific constellation of social support at work in the development of low back pain. *Journal of Occupational Health Psychology*, **7** (2), 130–140.

Elias, S.G., van Noord, P.A., Peeters, P.H., den Tonkelaar, I. & Grobbee, D.E. (2005) Childhood exposure to the 1944–1945 Dutch famine and subsequent female reproductive function. *Human Reproduction*, **20** (9), 2483–2488.

Eller, N.H., Netterstrom, B., Gyntelberg, F., *et al.* (2009) Work-related psychosocial factors and the development of ischemic heart disease: a systematic review. *Cardiology in Review*, **17** (2), 83–97.

Elvin-Novak, Y. (1999) Accompanied by guilt: modern motherhood the Swedish way. PhD thesis, Stockholm University.

Eriksson, M. & Lindström, B. (2005) Validity of Antonovsky's sense of coherence scale: a systematic review. *Journal of Epidemiology and Community Health*, **59** (6), 460–466.

European Agency for Safety and Health at Work (2008) Factsheet 78 – Work-related musculoskeletal disorders: prevention report. A summary. http://ew2007/osha.europa.eu. Last accessed 14 July 2010.

European Agency for Safety and Health at Work (2010) European Risk Observatory Report. OSH in figures: work-related musculoskeletal disorders in the EU – fact and figures. http://osha,europa.eu

European Commission (2007) Geographical mobility of citizens. Special Eurobarometer 281/Wave 67.1.

European Foundation for the Improvement of Living and Working Conditions (2005) Fourth European Working Conditions Survey. http://www.eurofound.europa.eu/ewco/surveys/ewcs2005/. Last accessed 14 July 2010.

European Foundation for the Improvement of Living and Working Conditions (2009) Drawing on experience – older women workers in Europe. http://www.eurofound.europa.eu

European Quality of Life Survey (2003) http://www.eurofound.europa.eu/publications/htmlfiles/ef04105 .htm. Last accessed 14 July 2010.

European Working Conditions Survey 2006. Office for Official Publications of the European Communities, Luxembourg.

Evans, G.W. (2003) A multimethodological analysis of cumulative risk and allostatic load among rural children. *Developmental Psychology*, **39** (5), 924–933.

Evans, G.W. (2004) The environment of childhood poverty. *American Psychologist*, **59** (2), 77–92.

Evans, G.W. & Kantrowitz, E. (2002) Socioeconomic status and health: the potential role of environmental risk exposure. *Annual Reviews of Publich Health*, **23**, 303–331.

Evans, P., Forte, D., Jacobs, C., *et al.* (2007) Cortisol secretory activity in older people in relation to positive and negative well-being. *Psychoneuroendocrinology*, **32**, 922–930.

Everson-Rose, S.A., Lewis, T.T., Karavolos, K., Dugan, S.A., Wesley, D. & Powell, L.H. (2009) Depressive symptoms and increased visceral fat in middle-aged women. *Psychosomatic Medicine*, **71**, 410–416.

Faragher, E.B., Cass, M. & Cooper, C.L. (2005) The relationship between job satisfaction and health: a meta-analysis. *Occupational and Environmental Medicine*, **62** (2), 105–112.

Faragher, E.B., Cooper, C.L. & Cartwright, S. (2004) A shortened stress evaluation tool. *Stress and Health*, **20** (4), 189–201.

Ferraro, K.F. & Su, Y.P. (2000) Physician-evaluated and self-reported morbidity for predicting disability. *American Journal of Public Health*, **90** (1), 103–108.

Fielden, S. & Cooper, C.L. (2002) Managerial stress: are women more at risk? In: *Gender, Work Stress and Health*, (eds D. L. Nelson & R. J. Burke), pp. 19–34. American Psychological Association, Washington, DC.

Francis, D.D., Diorio, J., Liu, D. & Meaney, M.J. (1999) Nongenomic transmission across generations in maternal behavior and stress responses in the rat. *Science*, **286** (5442), 1155–1158.

Frankenhaeuser, M. (1971) Behavior and circulating catecholamines. *Brain Research*, **31** (2), 241–262.

Frankenhaeuser, M. (1986) A psychobiological framework for research on human stress and coping. In: *Dynamics of Stress: Physiological, Psychological and Social Perspectives* (eds M.H. Appley & R. Trumbull), pp. 101–116. Plenum Press, New York.

Frankenhaeuser, M., Lundberg, U., Fredrikson, M., *et al.* (1989) Stress on and off the job as related to sex and occupational status in white-collar workers. *Journal of Organizational Behavior*, **10** (4), 321–346.

Frankenhaeuser, M., Nordheden, B., Myrsten, A.-L. & Post, B. (1971) Psychophysiological reactions to understimulation and overstimulation. *Acta Psychologica*, **35** (4), 298–308.

Fried, Y., Shirom, A & Cooper, C.L. (2008) Gender, age and tenure as moderators of work-related stressors' relationships with job performance. *Human Relations*, **61** (10), 1371–1398.

Friedman, M. & Rosenman, R.H. (1959) Association of specific overt behavior pattern with blood and cardiovascular findings; blood cholesterol level, blood clotting time, incidence of arcus senilis, and clinical coronary artery disease. *JAMA*, **169** (12), 1286–1296.

Friedman, M., Thoresen, C.E., Gill, J.J., *et al.* (1986) Alteration of type A behavior and its effect on cardiac recurrences in post myocardial infarction patients: summary results of the recurrent coronary prevention project. *American Heart Journal*, **112** (4), 653–665.

Frost, P., Kolstad, H.A. & Bonde, J.P. (2009) Shift work and the risk of ischemic heart disease — a systematic review of the epidemiological evidence. *Scandinavian Journal of Work, Environment & Health*, **35** (3), 163–179.

Gallo, L.C., Bogart, L.M., Vranceanu, A.M. & Walt, L.C. (2004) Job characteristics, occupational status, and ambulatory cardiovascular activity in women. *Annals of Behavioral Medicine*, **28** (1), 62–73.

Garde, A.H. & Hansen, A.M. (2005) Long-term stability of salivary cortisol. *Scandinavian Journal of Clinical & Laboratory Investigation*, **65** (5), 433–436.

Gatrell, C. (2005) *Hard Labour: The Sociology of Parenthood*. Open University Press, Maidenhead.

Gatrell, C. (2007) A fractional commitment? Part-time work and the maternal body. *International Journal of Human Resource Management*, **18** (3), 462–475.

Gatrell, C. & Cooper, C.L. (2008) Work–life balance: working for whom? *European Journal of International Management*, **2** (1), 71–86.

Geyer, S., Hemström, Ö., Peter, R. & Vågerö, D. (2006) Education, income and occupational class cannot be used interchangeably in social epidemiology. Empirical evidence against a common practice. *Journal of Epidemiological Community Health*, **60**, 804–810.

Gibson, C.B. (1995) Investigation of gender differences in leadership across four countries. *Journal of International Business Studies*, **26** (2), 255–279.

Gintzler, A.R. (1980) Endorphin-mediated increases in pain threshold during pregnancy. *Science*, **210** (4466), 193–195.

Gjerdingen, D., McGovern, P., Bekker, M., Lundberg, U. & Willemsen, T. (2000) Women's work roles and their impact on health, well-being and career: comparisons between the United States, Sweden, and The Netherlands. *Women and Health*, **31** (4), 1–20.

Goodman, E., McEwen, B.S., Huang, B., Dolan, L.M. & Adler, N. (2005) Social inequalities in biomarkers of cardiovascular risk in adolescence. *Psychosomatic Medicine*, **67** (1), 9–15.

Granges, G. & Littlejohn, G. (1993) Prevalence of myofascial pain syndrome in fibromyalgia. Muscle biopsy in fibromyalgia. *Journal of Musculoskeletal Pain*, **1** (3/4) 165.

Greenberg, P.E., Stiglin, L.E., Finkelstein, S.N. & Berndt, E.R. (1993) The economic burden of depression in 1990. *Journal of Clinical Psychiatry*, **54** (11), 405–418.

Grossi, G. (2008) Coping and emotional distress in a sample of Swedish unemployed. *Scandinavian Journal of Psychology*, **40** (3), 157–165.

Grønningsæter, H., Hytten, K., Skauli, G., Christensen, C.C. & Ursin, H. (1992) Improved health and coping by physical exercise or cognitive behavioural stress management training in a work environment. *Psychology and Health*, **7** (2), 147–163.

Gunnar, M. & Vazquez, D.M. (2001) Low cortisol and a flattening of expected daytime rhythm: potential indices of risk in human development. *Developmental Psychopathology*, **13** (3), 515–538.

Gustafsson, K., Lindfors, P., Aronsson, G. & Lundberg, U. (2008) Relationships between self-rating of recovery from work and morning salivary cortisol. *Journal of Occupational Health*, **50** (1), 24–30.

Hägg, G.M. (1991) Static work and myalgia – a new explanation model. In: *Electromyographical Kinesiology* (eds P.A. Andersson, D.J. Hobart, J.V. Danoff), pp. 115–199. Elsevier Science, Amsterdam.

Hansen, C.D. & Andersen, J.H. (2009) Sick at work – a risk factor for long-term sickness absence at a later date? *Journal of Epidemiology and Community Health*, **63** (5), 397–402.

Hansen, Å.M., Garde, A.H., Christensen, J.M., Eller, N.H. & Netterstrøm, B. (2001) Reference interval and biological variation of urinary epinephrine, norepinephrine, and cortisol in healthy subjects in Denmark. *Clinical Chemistry & Laboratory Medicine*, **39** (9), 842–849.

Hansen, Å.M., Garde, A.H., Skovgaard, L.T. & Christensen, J.M. (2001) Seasonal and biological variation of urinary epinephrine, norepinephrine, and cortisol in healthy women. *Clinica Chemica Acta*, **309** (1), 25–35.

Hansen, Å.M., Persson, R., Garde, A.H., Karlson, B. & Ørbæck, P. (2006) Diurnal profiles of salivary cortisol on workdays among construction workers versus white-collar workers. *Scandinavian Journal of Work, Environment & Health* (Suppl. 2), 22–26.

Hanson, M. (2004) Det flexibla arbetets villkor – om självförvaltandets kompetens. PhD thesis, Arbetslivsinstitutet, Pedagogiska institutionen, Stockholms universitet.

Härmä, M. & Kecklund, G. (2010) Shift work and health – how to proceed? *Scandinavian Journal of Work, Environment & Health*, **36** (2), 81–84.

Harris, K.F. & Matthews, K.A. (2004) Interactions between autonomic nervous system activity and endothelial function: a model for the development of cardiovascular disease. *Psychosomatic Medicine*, **66**, 153–164.

Harter, J.K., Schmidt, F.L. & Hays, T.L. (2002) Business-unit-level relationship between employee satisfaction, employee engagement, and business outcomes: a meta-analysis. *Journal of Applied Psychology*, **87** (2), 268–279.

Hartig, T. (2003) Restorative environments. *Journal of Environmental Psychology*, **23**, 103–107.

Hartig, T. (2008) Green space, psychological restoration, and health inequality. *Lancet*, **372** (9650), 1614–1615.

References **151**

Hartig, T. & Fransson, U. (2009) Leisure home ownership, access to nature, and health: a longitudinal study of urban residents in Sweden. *Environment and Planning*, **41** (1), 82–96.

Hartig, T., Catalano, R. & Ong, M. (2007) Cold summer weather, constrained restoration, and the use of antidepressants in Sweden. *Journal of Environmental Psychology*, **27** (2), 107–116.

Hawton, K. (2000) Sex and suicide. Gender differences in suicidal behaviour. *British Journal of Psychiatry*, **177**, 484–485.

Haynes, S.G., Feinleib, M., Levine, S., Scotch, N. & Kannel, W.B. (1978) The relationship of psychosocial factors to coronary heart disease in the Framingham study. II. Prevalence of coronary heart disease. *American Journal of Epidemiology*, **107** (5), 384–402.

Haynes, S.G., Levine, S., Scotch, N., Feinleib, M. & Kannel, W.B. (1978) The relationship of psychosocial factors to coronary heart disease in the Framingham study. I. Methods and risk factors. *American Journal of Epidemiology*, **107** (5), 362–383.

Health and Safety Executive (2009) http://www.hse.gov.uk/. Last accessed 9 July 2010.

Hellström, B. & Anderberg, U.M. (2003) Pain perception across the menstrual cycle phases in women with chronic pain. *Perceptual and Motor Skills*, **96** (1), 201–211.

Hellström, B. & Lundberg, U. (2000) Pain perception to the cold pressor test during the menstrual cycle in relation to estrogen levels and a comparison with men. *Integrative Physiological and Behavioral Science*, **35** (2), 132–141.

Hemingway, H. & Marmot, M. (1999) Psychosocial factors in the aetiology and prognosis of coronary heart disease: systematic review of prospective cohort studies. *British Medical Journal*, **318** (7196), 1460–1467.

Hemström, Ö. (2005) Health inequalities by wage income in Sweden: the role of work environment. *Social Science & Medicine*, **61** (3), 637–647.

Hendrix, K.H., Mayhan, S., Lackland, D.T. & Egan, B.M. (2005) Prevalence, treatment, and control of chest pain syndromes and associated risk factors in hypertensive patients. *American Journal of Hypertension*, **18** (8), 1026–1032.

Henneman, E., Somjen, G. & Carpenter, D.O. (1965) Excitability and inhibitability of motoneurons of different sizes. *Journal of Neurophysiology*, **28** (3), 599–620.

Henry, J.P. (1992) Biological basis of the stress response. *Integrative Physiological and Behavioral Science*, **27** (1), 66–83.

Henry, J.P. & Stephens, P.M. (1977) *Stress, Health, and the Social Environment. A Sociobiological Approach to Medicine*. Springer Verlag, New York.

Hillert, L., Åkerstedt, T., Lowden, A., *et al.* (2008) The effects of 884 MHz GSM wireless communication signals on headache and other symptoms: an experimental provocation study. *Bioelectromagnetics*, **29** (3), 185–196.

Hochschild, A. (1997) *The Time Bind: When Work Becomes Home and Home Becomes Work*. University of California Press, Berkeley.

Holmes, T.H. & Rahe, R.H. (1967) The social readjustment rating scale. *Journal of Psychosomatic Research*, **11** (2), 213–218.

Hoogendoorn, W.E., Bongers, P.M., de Vet, H.C.W., *et al.* (2001) Psychosocial work characteristics and psychological strain in relation to low back pain: results of a prospective cohort study. *Scandinavian Journal of Work, Environment & Health*, **27** (4), 258–267.

Hosie, P., Sevastos, P. & Cooper, C.L. (2007) *Happy-Performing Manager: The Impact of Affective Wellbeing and Intrinsic Job Satisfaction in the Workplace*. Edward Elgar, Cheltenham.

Hursti, T. (1994) Individual factors modifying chemotherapy related nausea and vomiting. PhD thesis, Karolinska Institutet, Stockholm.

ILO (2005) A global alliance against forced labour. Global report under the follow-up to the ILO Declaration on Fundamental Principles and Rights at Work. International Labour Office, Geneva.

Ishizaki, M., Nakagawa, H., Morikawa, Y., Honda, R., Yamada, Y., Kawakami, N., Japan Work Stress and Health (2008) Influence of job strain on changes in body mass index and waist circumference – 6-year longitudinal study. *Scandinavian Journal of Work, Environment & Health*, **34** (4), 288–296.

ISR (1995, 2000) Employee Satisfaction: Tracking European Trends. International Survey Research, London.

Ivancevich, J.M. & Matteson, M.T. (1987) Organizational level stress management interventions: a review and recommendations. *Journal of Organizational Behaviour Management*, **8** (2), 229–248.

Johansson, G. & Aronsson, G. (1984) Stress reactions in computerized administrative work. *Journal of Occupational Behaviour*, **5** (3), 159–181.

Johansson, H., Windhorst, U., Djupsjöbacka, M. & Passatore, M. (eds) (2003) *Chronic Work-Related Myalgia: Neuromuscular Mechanisms Behind Work-Related Chronic Muscle Pain Syndromes*. Gävle University Press, Gävle, Sweden.

Johnson, J.V. & Hall, E.M. (1988) Job strain, workplace social support and cardiovascular disease: a cross-sectional study of a random sample of the Swedish working population. *American Journal of Public Health*, **78** (10), 1336–1342.

Johnson, S., Cooper, C., Cartwright, S., Donald, I., *et al.* (2005) The experience of work-related stress across occupations. *Journal of Managerial Psychology*, **20** (2), 178–187.

Jonas, W. (2009) Mother and newborn adaptations after birth. Influence of administration of oxytocin an epidural analgesia during labour. PhD thesis, Karolinska Institute, Sweden.

Kahn, R.L. (1991) The forms of women's work. In: *Women, Work and Health: Stress and Opportunities* (eds M. Frankenhaeuser, U. Lundberg & M.A. Chesney), pp. 65–83. Plenum Press, New York.

Kaplan, J.R., Chen, H. & Manuck, S.B. (2009) The relationship between social status and atherosclerosis in male and female monkeys as revealed by meta-analysis. *American Journal of Primatology*, **71** (9), 732–741.

Karasek, R.A. (1979) Job demands, job decision latitude, and mental strain: implications for job redesign. *Administrative Science Quarterly*, **24** (2), 285–308.

Karasek, R.A. & Theorell, T. (1990) *Healthy Work: Stress, Productivity and the Reconstruction of Working Life*, pp. 89–103. Basic Books, New York.

Kawachi, I. & Kennedy B.P. (2002) *The Health of Nations: Why Inequality is Harmful to Your Health*. New York Academy of Science, vol. 896. The New Press, New York.

Kempermann, G., Kuhn, H.G. & Gage, F.H. (1997) More hippocampal neurons in adult mice living in an enriched environment. *Nature*, **386** (6624), 493–495.

Kentää, G. (2001) Overtraining, staleness, and burnout in sports. PhD thesis, Stockholm University, Sweden.

Kessler, R.C. & Frank, R.G. (1997) The impact of psychiatric disorders on work loss days. *Psychological Medicine*, **27**, 179–190.

Kiecolt-Glaser, J.K., Marucha, P.T., Malarkey, W.B., Mercado, A.M. & Glaser, R. (1995) Slowing of wound healing by psychological stress. *Lancet*, **346** (8984), 1194–1196.

Kimbrough, E., Magyari, T., Langenberg, P., Chesney, M. & Berman, B. (2010) Mindfulness intervention for child abuse survivors. *Journal of Clinical Psychology*, **66**, 17–33.

Kivimäki, M., Ferrie, E., Brunner, E., *et al.* (2005) FRCP Justice at work and reduced risk of coronary heart disease among employees: The Whitehall II Study. *Archives of Internal Medicine*, **165**, 2245–2251.

Kivimäki, M., Head, J., Ferrie, J., *et al.* (2005) Working while ill as a risk factor for serious coronary events: The Whitehall II Study. *American Journal of Public Health*, **95** (1), 98–102.

Kivimäki, M., Leino-Arjas, P., Kaila-Kangas, L., *et al.* (2004) A review of fibromyalgia. *American Journal of Managed Care*, **10**, 794–800.

Kivimäki, M., Vahtera, J., Ferrie, J.E., *et al.* (2001) Organisational downsizing and musculoskeletal problems in employees: a prospective study. *Occupational and Environmental Medicine*, **58** (12), 811–817.

Kivimäki, M., Vahtera, J., Pentti, J., *et al.* (2000) Factors underlying the effect of organisational downsizing on health of employees: longitudinal cohort study. *British Medical Journal*, **320** (7240), 971–975.

Kivimäki, M., Vahtera, J., Virtanen, M., *et al.* (2003) Temporary employment and risk of overall and cause-specific mortality. *American Journal of Epidemiology*, **158** (7), 663–668.

Kivimäki, M., Virtanen, M., Elovainio, M., *et al.* (2006) Work stress in the etiology of coronary heart disease–a meta-analysis. *Scandinavian Journal of Work, Environment & Health*, **32** (6), 431–442.

Klumb, P., Hoppmann, C. & Staats, M. (2006) Work hours affect spouse's cortisol secretion – for better and for worse. *Psychosomatic Medicine*, **68** (5), 742–746.

Knapp, M. (2009) Mental ill health: cost implications. In: *Mental Capital and Wellbeing* (eds Cooper, C., Goswami, U. & Sahakian, B.J.), pp. 515–529. Wiley-Blackwell, Oxford.

Knardahl, S. (2002) Psychophysiological mechanisms of pain in computer work: the blood vessel–nociceptor interaction hypothesis. *Work & Stress*, **16** (2), 179–189.

Kornitzer, M., DeSmet, P., Sans, S., *et al.* (2006) Job stress and major coronary events: results from the Job Stress, Absenteeism and Coronary Heart Disease in Europe study. *European Journal of Cardiovascular Prevention & Rehabilitation*, **13** (5), 695–704.

Krantz, G., Berntsson, L. & Lundberg, U. (2005) Total workload, work stress and perceived symptoms in Swedish male and female white-collar employees. *European Journal of Public Health*, **15** (2), 209–214.

Krantz, G., Forsman, M. & Lundberg, U. (2004) Consistency in physiological stress responses and electromyographic activity during induced stress exposure in women and men. *Integrative Physiological and Behavioral Science*, **39** (2), 105–118.

Kristensen, T. (1991) Sickness absence and work strain among Danish slaughterhouse workers: an analysis of absence from work regarded as coping behavior. *Social Science Medicine*, **32** (1), 15–27.

Kristensen, T., Borg, V. & Hannerz, H. (2002) Socioeconomic status and psychosocial work environment: results from a Danish national study. *Scandinavian Journal of Public Health*, **30** (59, Suppl), 41–48.

Kristenson, K. (1998) The LiVicordia study. Possible causes for the differences in coronary heart disease mortality between Lithuania and Sweden. PhD thesis, Department of Health and Environment, Linköping University, Sweden.

Kristenson, M., Eriksen, H.R., Sluiter, J.K., Starke, D. & Ursin, H. (2004) Psychobiological mechanisms of socioeconomic differences in health. *Social Science & Medicine*, **58** (8), 1511–1522.

Kristenson, M., Orth-Gomér, K., Kucienskiene, Z., *et al.* (1998) Attenuated cortisol response to a standardised stress test in Lithuanian vs Swedish men: the LiVicordia study. *International Journal of Behavioral Medicine*, **5** (1), 17–30.

Kuiper, J.I., van der Beek, A.J. & Meijman, T.F. (1998) Psychosomatic complaints and unwinding of sympathoadrenal activation after work. *Stress Medicine*, **14** (1), 7–12.

Kumlin, L., Latscha, G., Orth-Gomér, K., *et al.* (2001) Marital status and cardiovascular risk in French and Swedish automotive industry workers – cross sectional results from the Renault–Volvo Coeur study. *Journal of Internal Medicine*, **249** (4), 315–323.

Kuper, H. & Marmot, M. (2003) Job strain, job demands, decision latitude, and risk of coronary heart disease within the Whitehall II study. *Journal of Epidemiology & Community Health*, **57** (2), 147–153.

Kuruba, R., Hattiangady, B. & Shetty, A.K. (2009) Hippocampal neurogenesis and neural stem cells in temporal lobe epilepsy. *Epilepsy & Behaviour*, **14** (Suppl. 1), 65–73.

Kyffin, R.G.E., Goldacre, M.J. & Gill, M. (2004) Mortality rates and self reported health: database analysis by English local authority area. *British Medical Journal*, **329** (7471), 887–888.

Lager, A. & Bremberg, S. (2009) Association between labour market trends and trends in young people's mental health in ten European countries 1983–2005. *BMC Public Health*, **9**, 325.

Lammi-Taskula, J. (2006) Nordic men on parental leave: can the welfare state change gender relations? In: *Politicising Parenthood in Scandinavia, Gender Relations in Welfare States* (eds A. Ellingsæater & A. Leira), pp. 79–101. Policy Press, Bristol.

Laursen, B., Jensen, B.R., Garde, A.H. & Jørgenson, A.H. (2002) Effect of mental and physical demands on muscular activity during the use of a computer mouse and a keyboard. *Scandinavian Journal of Work, Environment & Health*, **28** (4), 215–221.

Lee, I.M., Sesso, H.D. & Paffenberger, R.S. (2000) Physical activity and coronary heart disease risk in men: does the duration of exercise episodes predict risk? *Circulation*, **102** (9), 981–986.

Leino, P. & Magni, G. (1993) Depressive and distress symptoms as predictors of low back pain, neck shoulder pain, and other musculoskeletal morbidity: a 10-year follow-up of metal industry employees. *Pain*, **53** (1), 89–94.

Leserman, J. (2008) Role of depression, stress, and trauma in HIV disease progression. *Psychosomatic Medicine*, **70** (5), 539–545.

Levi, L. (1990) Occupational stress. Spice of life or kiss of death? *American Psychologist*, **45** (10), 1142–1145.

Lewis, S. & Cooper, C.L. (2005) *Work–Life Integration: Case Studies in Organizational Change*. John Wiley & Sons, Chichester.

Lewis, S., Gambles, R., & Rapoport, R. (2007) The constraints of a 'work–life balance' approach: an international perspective. *International Journal of Human Resource Management*, **18** (3), 360–372.

Li, L., Power, C., Kelly, S. & Kirschbaum, C. (2007) Life-time socio-economic position and cortisol patterns in mid-life. *Psychoneuroendocrinology*, **32** (7), 824–833.

Lichtman, J.H., Bigger, J.T., Jr, Blumenthal, J.A., *et al.* (2008) Depression and coronary heart disease: recommendations for screening, referral, and treatment: a science advisory from the American Heart Association Prevention Committee of the Council on Cardiovascular Nursing, Council on Clinical Cardiology, Council on Epidemiology and Prevention, and Interdisciplinary Council on Quality of Care and Outcomes Research: endorsed by the American Psychiatric Association. *Circulation*, **118** (17), 1768–1775.

Lindfors, P. & Lundberg, U. (2002) Is low cortisol release and indicator of positive health? *Stress and Health*, **18** (4), 153–160.

Lindfors, P., Lundberg, O. & Lundberg, U. (2006) Allostatic load and clinical risk as related to sense of coherence in middle-aged women. *Psychosomatic Medicine*, **68** (5), 801–807.

Linton, S. (ed.) (2002) *Avenues for the Prevention of Chronic Musculoskeletal Pain and Disability*. Elsevier Science, New York.

Llabre, M.M. & Hadi, F. (2009) War-related exposure and psychological distress as predictors of health and sleep: a longitudinal study of Kuwaiti children. *Psychosomatic Medicine*, **71**, 776–783.

Luecken, L.J., Suarez, E.C., Kuhn, C.M., *et al.* (1997) Stress in employed women: impact of marital status and children at home on neurohormone. *Psychosomatic Medicine*, **59** (4), 352–359.

Lundberg, O. & Fritzell, J. (1994) Income distribution, income change, and health. On the importance of absolute and relative income for health status in Sweden. In: *The Effects of Economic Changes on Social Welfare and Health* (eds L. Levin, L. McMahon & E. Ziglio). World Health Organization, Copenhagen.

Lundberg, U. (1984) Human psychobiology in Scandinavia: II Psychoneuro-endocrinology, human stress and coping processes. *Scandinavian Journal of Psychology*, **25** (3), 214–226.

Lundberg, U. (1996) The influence of paid and unpaid work on psychophysiological stress responses of men and women. *Journal of Occupational Health Psychology*, **1** (2), 117–130.

Lundberg, U. (2007) Workplace stress. In: *Encyclopedia of Stress* (ed. G. Fink), pp. 871–875. Academic Press, San Diego.

Lundberg, U. (2009a) Stress, health and illness as related to work and gender. In: *How Stress Influences Musculoskeletal Disorders* (ed. K.-A. Lindgren), pp. 11–15. Orton Foundation, Helsinki.

Lundberg, U. (2009b) Physiological stress reactions and musculoskeletal disorders. In: *How Stress Influences Musculoskeletal Disorders* (ed. K.-A. Lindgren), pp. 21–25. Orton Foundation, Helsinki.

Lundberg, U. & Forsman, L. (1980) Consistency in catecholamine and cortisol excretion patterns over experimental conditions. *Pharmacology, Biochemistry and Behavior*, **12** (3), 449–452.

Lundberg, U. & Frankenhaeuser, M. (1999) Stress and workload of men and women in high ranking positions. *Journal of Occupational Health Psychology*, **4** (2), 142–151.

Lundberg, U. & Hellström, B. (2002) Workload and morning salivary cortisol in women. *Work & Stress*, **16** (4), 356–363.

Lundberg, U. & Johansson, G. (2000) Stress and health risks in repetitive work and supervisory monitoring work. In: *Engineering Psychophysiology: Issues and Applications* (eds R. Backs & W. Boucsein), pp. 339–359. Lawrence Erlbaum, New Jersey.

Lundberg, U. & Lindfors, P. (2002) Psychophysiological reactions to telework in female and male white-collar workers. *Journal of Occupational Health Psychology*, **7** (4), 354–364.

Lundberg, U. & Palm, K. (1989) Total workload and catecholamine excretion of families with preschool children. *Work & Stress*, **3** (3), 255–260.

Lundberg, U., Forsman, M., Zachau, G., *et al.* (2002) Effects of experimentally induced mental and physical stress on trapezius motor unit recruitment in the trapezius muscle. *Work & Stress*, **16** (2), 166–178.

Lundberg, U., Granqvist, M., Hansson, T., Magnusson, M. & Wallin, L. (1989) Psychological and physiological stress responses during repetitive work at an assembly line. *Work & Stress*, **3** (2), 143–153.

Lundberg, U., Kadefors, R., Melin, B., *et al.* (1994) Psychophysiological stress and EMG activity of the trapezius muscle. *International Journal of Behavioural Medicine*, **1** (4), 354–370.

Lundberg, U., Mårdberg, B. & Frankenhaeuser, M. (1994) The total workload of male and female white collar workers as related to age, occupational level, and number of children. *Scandinavian Journal of Psychology*, **35** (4), 315–327.

Lupien, S.J., King, S., Meaney, M.J. & McEwen, B.S. (2000) Child's stress hormone levels correlate with mother's socioeconomic status and depressive state. *Biological Psychiatry*, **48** (10), 976–980.

Mackenbach, J.P. (2002) Income inequality and population health. Evidence favouring a negative correlation between income inequality and life expectancy has disappeared. *British Medical Journal*, **324**, 1–2.

Mackenbach, J.P., Bakker, M.J. & European Network on Interventions and Policies to Reduce Inequalities in Health (2003) Tackling socioeconomic inequalities in health: analysis of European experiences. *Lancet*, **362** (9393), 1409–1414.

Maloney, E.M., Boneva, R., Nater, U.M. & Reeves, W.C. (2009) Chronic fatigue syndrome and high allostatic load: results from a population-based case-control study in Georgia. *Psychosomatic Medicine*, **71** (5), 549–556.

Marmot, M. (2004) *Status Syndrome: How Your Social Standing Directly Affects Your Health and Life Expectancy*. Bloomsbury, London.

Marmot, M. (Chair, Commission on the Social Determinants of Health) (2008) Closing the Gap in a Generation: Health Equity through Action on the Social Determinants of Health. World Health Organization, Geneva.

Marmot, M. & Shipley, M.J. (1996) Do socioeconomic differences in mortality persist after retirement? 25 year follow up of civil servants from the first Whitehall study. *British Medical Journal*, **313** (7066), 1177–1180.

Marmot, M. & Wilkinson, R.G. (eds) (2006) *Social Determinants of Health*, 2nd edn. Oxford University Press, Oxford, UK.

Marmot, M., Rose, G., Shipley, M. & Hamilton, P.J. (1978) Employment grade and coronary heart disease in British civil servants. *Journal of Epidemiology and Community Health*, **32** (4), 244–249.

Marras, W.S., Davis, K.G., Heaney, C.A., Maronitis, A.B. & Allread, W.G. (2000) The influence of psychosocial stress, gender, and personality on mechanical loading of the lumbar spine. *Spine*, **25** (23), 3045–3054.

Marucha, P.T., Kiecolt-Glaser J.K. & Favagehi, M. (1998) Mucosal wound healing is impaired by examination stress. *Psychosomatic Medicine*, **60** (3), 362–365.

Mason, J.W., Wang, S., Yehuda, R., *et al.* (2002) Marked lability in urinary cortisol levels in subgroups of combat veterans with posttraumatic stress disorder during an intensive exposure treatment program. *Psychosomatic Medicine*, **64** (2), 238–246.

Matthews, K.A., Räikkönen, K., Everson, S.A., *et al.* (2000) Do the daily experiences of healthy men and women vary according to occupational prestige and work strain? *Psychosomatic Medicine*, **62** (3), 346–353.

McEwen, B.S. (1998) Stress, adaptation and disease: allostasis and allostatic load. *New England Journal of Medicine*, **840**, 33–44.

McEwen, B.S. & Lasley, E.N. (2002) *The End of Stress as We Know it*. Joseph Henry Press, Washington, DC.

McLeod, J. (2001) *Counselling in the Workplace. The Facts. A Systematic Study of the Research Evidence*. British Association for Counselling and Psychotherapy, Rugby.

Meaney, M.J. (2001) Maternal care, gene expression, and the transmission of individual differences in stress reactivity across generations. *Annual Review of Neuroscience*, **24**, 1161–1192.

Mehlum, I.S., Kristensen, P., Kjuus, H. & Wergeland, E. (2008) Are occupational factors important determinants of socioeconomic inequalities in musculoskeletal pain? *Scandinavian Journal of Work, Environment & Health*, **34** (4), 250–259.

Melin, B. & Lundberg, U. (1997) A biopsychosocial approach to work-stress and musculoskeletal disorders. *Journal of Psychophysiology*, **11** (3), 238–247.

Melin, B., Lundberg, U., Söderlund, J. & Granqvist, M. (1999) Psychophysiological stress reactions of male and female assembly workers: a comparison between two different forms of work organizations. *Journal of Organizational Behavior*, **20**, 47–61.

Menkes, M.S., Matthews, K.A., Krantz, D.S., *et al.* (1989) Cardiovascular reactivity to the cold pressor test as a predictor of hypertension. *Hypertension*, **14** (5), 524–530.

Meyer, K., Niemann, S. & Abel, T. (2004) Gender differences in physical activity and fitness – association with self-reported health and health-relevant attitudes in a middle-aged Swiss urban population. *Journal of Public Health*, **12** (4), 283–290.

Miller, G. (2009) Sleeping to reset overstimulated synapses. *Science*, **324** (5923), 22.

Miller, G.E., Chen, E. & Zhou, E.S. (2007) If it goes up, must it come down? Chronic stress and the hypothalamic–pituitary–adrenocortical axis in humans. *Psychological Bulletin*, **133** (1), 25–45.

Miller, G.E., Cohen, S., Pressman, S., Barkin, A., Rabin, B.S. & Treanor, J.J. (2004) Psychological stress and antibody response to influenza vaccination: when is the critical period of stress, and how does it get inside the body? *Psychosomatic Medicine*, **66** (2), 215–223.

Miranda, H., Viikari-Juntura, E., Punnet, L. & Riihimäki, H. (2008) Occupational loading, health behavior and sleep disturbance as predictors of low-back pain. *Scandinavian Journal of Work, Environment & Health*, **34** (6), 411–419.

Moskowitz, J.T. (2003) Positive affect predicts lower risk of AIDS mortality. *Psychosomatic Medicine*, **65** (4), 620–626.

Muller, A. (2002) Education, income inequality, and mortality: a multiple regression analysis. *British Medical Journal*, **324** (7328), 23–25.

Naylor, A.S., Persson, A.I., Eriksson, P.S., Jonsdottir, I.H. & Thorlin, T. (2005) Extended voluntary running inhibits exercise-induced adult hippocampal progenitor proliferation in the spontaneously hypertensive rat. *Journal of Neurophysiology*, **93** (5), 2406–2414.

Netterstrøm, B., Kristensen, T.S. & Sjøl, A. (2006) Psychological job demands increase the risk of ischaemic heart disease: a 14-year cohort study of employed Danish men. *European Journal of Cardiovascular Prevention & Rehabilitation*, **13** (3), 414–420.

Niedhammer, I., Goldberg, M., Leclerc, A., Bugel, I. & David, S. (1998) Psychological factors at work and subsequent depressive symptoms in the Gazel cohort. *Scandinavian Journal of Work, Environment and Health*, **24** (3), 197–205.

Nieman, D.C. (1998) *The Exercise–Health Connection*. Human Kinetics Publishers, Champaign, IL.

NIOSH (2002) The Changing Organization of Work and the Safety and Health of Working People. National Institute of Occupational Safety and Health, Publ. No. 116.

Nordander, C., Ohlsson, K., Balogh, I., Rylander, L., Pålsson, B. & Skerfving, S. (1999) Fish processing work: the impact of two sex dependent exposure profiles on musculoskeletal health. *Occupational and Environmental Medicine*, **56** (4), 256–264.

Nordander, C., Ohlsson, K., Balogh, I., *et al.* (2008) Gender differences in workers with identical repetitive industrial tasks: exposure and musculoskeletal disorders. *International Archives of Occupational and Environmental Health*, **81** (8), 939–947.

Nordlund, A. & Waddell, G. (2000) Samhällets totala kostnader för ont i ryggen. In: *Ont i Ryggen, ont i Nacken: En Evidensbaserad Kunskapssammanställning*, Vol. II (eds E. Jonsson & A. Nachemson), pp. 297–309. Statens beredning for medicinsk utvärdering, Stockholm.

Nyklíček, I. & Kuijpers, K.F. (2008) Effects of mindfulness-based stress reduction intervention on psychological well-being and quality of life: is increased mindfulness indeed the mechanism? *Annals of Behavioral Medicine*, **35** (3), 331–340.

Öhman, A. & Soares, J.J.F. (1994) "Unconscious anxiety": phobic responses to masked stimuli. *Journal of Abnormal Psychology*, **103** (2), 231–240.

Östlin, P. (2004) Priorities for research to take forward the health equity policy agenda. Report from the WHO Task Force on Health System Research Priorities for Equity in Health.

Östlin, P. & Diderichsen, F. (2001) Equity-oriented national strategy for public health in Sweden: a case study. Policy Learning Curve Series number 1, updated version. World Health Organization, Brussels.

Opotowsky, A.R., McWilliams, J.M. & Cannon, C.P. (2007) Women continue to fare worse than men in treatment for heart attack and congestive heart failure. *Journal of General Internal Medicine*, **22**, 55–61.

Ostry, A.S., Kelly, S., Demers, P.A., Mustard, C. & Hertzman, C. (2003) A comparison between the effort–reward imbalance and demand control models. *BMC Public Health*, **3**, 10.

Paganetto, L. (ed.) (2004) *Knowledge Economy, Information Technologies and Growth*. Ashgate, Aldershot.

Palmer, S., Cooper, C.L. & Thomas, K. (2003) *Creating a Balance: Managing Stress*. British Library, London.

Parent-Thirion, A., Macias, E.F., Hurley, J. & Vermeylen, G. (2007) Fourth European Conditions Survey. European Foundation for the Improvement of Working and Living Conditions, Dublin.

Park, J., Cho, Y., Yi, K-H., Rhee, K-Y., Kim, Y. & Moon, Y-H. (1999) Unexpected natural deaths among Korean workers. *Journal of Occupational Health*, **41** (4), 238–243.

Park, J., Kim, Y., Cho, Y., *et al.* (2001) Regular overtime and cardiovascular functions. *Industrial Health*, **39** (3), 244–249.

Park, J., Kim, Y., Chung, H.K. & Hisanaga, N. (2001) Long working hours and subjective fatigue symptoms. *Industrial Health*, **39** (33), 250–254.

Passmore, J. & Anagnos, J. (2009) Organizational coaching and mentoring. In: *The Oxford Handbook of Organizational Wellbeing* (eds S. Cartwright & C. L. Cooper). Oxford University Press, Oxford.

Peeters, F., Nicholson, N.A. & Berkhof, J. (2003) Cortisol responses to daily events in major depressive disorder. *Psychosomatic Medicine*, **65** (5), 836–841.

Peiper, S. & Brosschot, J.F. (2005) Prolonged stress-related cardiovascular activation: Is there any? *Annals of Behavioral Medicine*, **30** (2), 91–103.

Pejtersen, J.H. & Kristensen T.S. (2009) The development of the psychosocial work environment in Denmark from 1997 to 2005. *Scandinavian Journal of Work, Environment & Health*, **35** (4), 284–293.

Peña-Casas, R. & Pochet, P. (2009) *Convergence and Divergence of Working Conditions in Europe: 1990–2005*. European Foundation for the Improvement of Living and Working Conditions, Dublin.

Penninx, B.W., Rejeski, W.J., Pandya, J., *et al.* (2002) Exercise and depressive symptoms: a comparison of aerobic and resistance exercise effects on emotional and physical function in older persons with high and low depressive symptomatology. *Journal of Gerontology*, **57** (2), 124–132.

Persell, S.D., Maviglia, S., Bates, D.W. & Ayanian, J.Z. (2005) Management of chest pain differs by sex and race. *Journal of General Internal Medicine*, **20**, 123–130.

Persson, R., Garde, A.H., Hansen, Å.M., *et al.* (2008) Seasonal variation in human salivary cortisol concentration. *Chronobiology International*, **25** (6), 923–937.

Petitti, D. (2009) Hormone replacement therapy and coronary heart disease: results of randomized trials. *Progress in Cardiovascular Diseases*, **46** (3), 231–238.

Petzke, F., Clauw, D.J., Ambrose, K., Khine, A. & Gracely, R.H. (2003) Increased pain sensitivity in fibromyalgia: effects of stimulus type and mode of presentation. *Pain*, **105** (3), 403–413.

Pollard, T.M. (1995) Use of cortisol as a stress marker: practical and theoretical problems. *American Journal of Human Biology*, **7** (2), 265–274.

Pressman, S.D., Matthews, K.A., Cohen, S., *et al.* (2009) Association of enjoyable leisure activities with psychological and physical well-being. *Psychosomatic Medicine*, **71**, 725–732.

Preussner, J.C., Hellhammer, D.H. & Kirschbaum, C. (1999) Burnout, perceived stress, and cortisol responses to awakening. *Psychosomatic Medicine*, **61** (2), 197–204.

Preussner, M., Hellhammer, D.H., Preussner, J.P. & Lupien, S.J. (2003) Self-reported depressive symptoms and stress levels in healthy young men: associations with the cortisol response to awakening. *Psychosomatic Medicine*, **65** (1), 92–99.

Price, D.D. (2000) Psychological and neural mechanisms of the affective dimension of pain. *Science*, **288** (5472), 1769–1772.

PricewaterhouseCoopers (2008) *Building the Case for Wellness*. PricewaterhouseCoopers, London.

Räikkönen, K., Matthews, K.A., Sutton-Tyrrell, K. & Kuller, L.H. (2004) Trait anger and the metabolic syndrome predict progression of carotid atherosclerosis in healthy middle-aged women. *Psychosomatic Medicine*, **66**, 903–908.

Rayner, C., Hoel, H. & Cooper, C.L. (2002) *Workplace Bullying: What We Know, Who Is to Blame and What Can We Co?* Taylor & Francis, London.

Rhodes, S.R. & Steers, R.M. (1990) *Managing Employee Absenteeism.* Addison-Wesley, Reading, MA.

Richards, S.C. & Scott, D.L. (2002) Prescribed exercise in people with fibromyalgia: parallel group randomised controlled trial. *British Medical Journal*, **325** (7357), 185–187.

Richter, P.G., Rau, R. & Mühlpfordt, D. (eds) (2007) *Arbeit und Gesundheit. Zum aktuellen Stand in einem Forschungs- und Praxisfeld.* Pabst, Lengerich.

Riedmann, A., Bielenski, H., Szczurowska, T. & Wagner, A. (2006) Working time and work–life balance in European companies. Office for Official Publications of the European Communities, Luxembourg.

Riley, J.L., Robinson, M.E., Wise, E.A., Myers, C.D. & Fillingim, R.B. (1998) Sex differences in the perception of noxious experimental stimuli: a meta-analysis. *Pain*, **74**, 181–187.

Rissén, D. (2006) Repetitive and monotonous work among women: psychophysiological and subjective stress reactions, muscle activity and neck and shoulder pain. PhD thesis, Department of Psychology, Stockholm University.

Rissén, D., Melin, B., Sandsjö, L., Dohns, I. & Lundberg, U. (2002) Psychophysiological stress reactions, trapezius muscle activity and neck and shoulder pain among female cashiers; before and after a work re-organization. *Work & Stress*, **16** (2), 127–137.

Rissler, A. (1977) Stress reactions at work and after work during a period of quantitative overload. *Ergonomics*, **20**, 577–580.

Riva, R., Mork, P.J., Westgaard, R.H., Rø, M. & Lundberg, U. (2010) Fibromyalgia syndrome is associated with hypocortisolism. *International Journal of Behavioral Medicine*, **17** (3), 223–233.

Robertson, I. & Flint-Taylor, J. (2009) Leadership, psychological wellbeing and organizational outcomes. In: *The Oxford Handbook of Organizational Wellbeing* (eds S. Cartwright & C. L. Cooper). Oxford University Press, Oxford.

Robertson Cooper (2008) *Cost and Benefit Analysis of Wellbeing.* RCL, Manchester.

Rogers, M.A.M., Blumberg, N.B., Saint, S.K. *et al.* (2006) Women with atherosclerosis and high cholesterol receive less intense cholesterol management than men. *American Heart Journal*, **152**, 1028–1034.

Romeri, E., Baker, A. & Griffiths, C. (2006) Mortality by deprivation and cause of death in England and Wales, 1999–2003. *Health Statistics Quarterly*, **32**, 19–34.

Rosener, J.B. (1990) Ways women lead. *Harvard Business Review*, **63** (6), 119–125.

Rosenman, R.H. & Chesney, M.A. (1980) The relationships of Type A behavior to coronary heart disease. *Activitas Nervosa Superior*, **22**, 1–45.

Rosenman, R.H., Brand, R.J., Sholtz, R.I. & Friedman, M. (1976) Multivariate prediction of coronary heart disease during 8.5 years follow-up in the Western Collaborative Group Study. *American Journal of Cardiology*, **37** (6), 903–910.

Rosmond, R. & Björntorp, P. (2000) Occupational status, cortisol secretory pattern, and visceral obesity in middle-aged men. *Obesity Research*, **8** (6), 445–450.

Rotter, J.B. (1966) Generalized expectancies for internal versus external control of reinforcement. *Psychological Monographs*, **80** (1), 1–28.

Ryff, C.D. & Singer, B.H. (1998) The contours of positive human health. *Psychological Inquiry*, **9** (1), 1–28.

Sachar, E.J. & Baron, M. (1979) The biology of affective disorders. *Annual Review of Neuroscience*, **2**, 505–518.

Sainsbury Centre for Mental Health (2007) *Estimate Annual Costs to UK Employers of Mental Ill Health.* Sainsbury Centre for Mental Health, London.

Sapolsky, R. (1996) Why stress is bad for your brain. *Science*, **273** (5276), 749–750.

Sapolsky, R. (1998) *Why Zebras Don't Get Ulcers: An Updated Guide to Stress, Stress-Related Disease and Coping.* WH Freeman and Co., New York.

Sapolsky, R. (2005) The influence of social hierarchy on primate health. *Science*, **308** (5722), 648–652.

Schernhammer, E.S. & Colditz, G.A. (2004) Suicide rates among physicians: a quantitative and gender assessment (meta-analysis). *American Journal of Psychiatry*, **161** (12), 2295–2302.

Schleifer, L.M. & Ley, R. (1994) End-tidal PCO_2 as an index of psychophysiological activity during VDT data-entry work and relaxation. *Ergonomics*, **37** (2), 245–254.

Schnall, P.L., Dobson, M. & Rosskam, E. (eds) (2009) *Unhealthy Work: Causes, Consequences, Cures.* Baywook Publishing Company Inc., Amityville, New York.

Seeman, T.E., McEwen, B.S., Singer, B.H., Albert, M.S. & Rowe, J.W. (1997) Increase in urinary cortisol excretion and memory declines: MacArthur studies of successful aging. *The Journal of Clinical Endocrinology & Metabolism*, **82** (8), 2458–2465.

Seligman, M.E.P. (1975) *Helplessness: On Depression, Development, and Death.* W.H. Freeman, San Francisco.

Selye, H. (1956) *The Stress of Life.* McGraw-Hill, New York.

Semmer, N.K., Tschan, F., Meier, L.L., Facchin, S. & Jacobshagen, N. (2010) Illegitimate tasks and counterproductive work behavior. *Applied Psychology*, **59** (1), 70–96.

Shibuya, K., Hashimoto, H. & Yano, E. (2002) Individual income, income distribution, and self rated health in Japan: cross sectional analysis of nationally representative sample. *British Medical Journal*, **324** (16), 16–19.

Shirom, A., Gilboa, S.S., Fried, Y. & Cooper, C.L. (2008) Gender, age and tenure as moderators of work-related stressors' relationships with job performance. *Human Relations*, **61** (10), 1371–1398.

Siegrist, J. (1996) Adverse health effects of high effort–low reward conditions at work. *Journal of Occupational Health Psychology*, **1** (1), 27–43.

Siegrist, J. (2008) Effort–reward imbalance and health in a globalized economy. *Scandinavian Journal of Work, Environment & Health*, **34** (Special Issue 6), 163–168.

Silverstein, B. & Adams, D. (2007) Work-related musculoskeletal disorders of the neck, back, and upper extremity in Washington State, 1997–2005. Technical Report Number 40-11. Safety & Health Assessment & Research for Prevention (SHARP) and Washington State Department of Labor and Industries, Olympia, WA.

Silverstein, B., Fan, Z.J., Smith, C.K., *et al.* (2009) Gender adjustment or stratification in discerning upper extremity musculoskeletal disorder risk? *Scandinavian Journal of Work, Environment & Health*, **35** (2), 113–126.

Simon, A., Dimberg, L., Levenson, J. *et al.* (1997) Comparison of cardiovascular risk profile between male employees of two automotive companies in France and Sweden. *European Journal of Epidemiology*, **13** (8), 885–891.

Simon, R.W. (1995) Gender differences in reference groups, self-evaluations, and emotional experience among employed married parents. *Advances in Group Processes* (eds B. Markovsky, K. Heimer & J. O'Brien), vol. 12, pp. 19–50. JAI Press, Greenwich, CT.

Sjöholm, Å. (2007) Stark koppling mellan bukfetma och socioekonomiska faktorer. (Strong association between abdominal fat and socioeconomic factors). *Läkartidningen*, **104**, 3862–3866.

Sora, B., Caballer, A., Peir, J.M. & de Witte, H. (2009) Job insecurity climate's influence on employees' job attitudes: evidence from two European countries. *European Journal of Work and Organizational Psychology*, **18** (2), 125–147.

Sparrow, P. & Cooper, C.L. (2003) *The Employment Relationship.* Elsevier, London.

Spector, P., Allen, T., Cooper, C.L., Lapierre, L. & Poelmans, S. (2007) Cross-national differences in relationships of work demands, job satisfaction and turnover intentions with work-family conflict. *Personnel Psychology*, **60** (4), 805–835.

Spiegel, K., Knutson, K., Leproult, R. Tasali, E. & Van Couter, E. (2005) Sleep loss: a novel risk factor for insulin resistance and Type 2 diabetes. *Journal of Applied Physiology*, **99** (5), 2008–2019.

Stansfeld, S. & Candy, B. (2006) Psychosocial work environment and mental health – a meta-analytic review. *Scandinavian Journal of Work, Environment and Health*, **32** (6), 443–462.

Starkman, M.N., Gebrarski, S., Berent, S. & Schteingart, D. (1992) Hippocampal formation volume, memory dysfunction, and cortisol levels in patients with Cushing's syndrome. *Biological Psychiatry*, **32** (9), 756–765.

Starkman, M.N., Giordani, B., Berent, S., Schork, M.A. & Schteingart, D.E. (2001) Elevated cortisol levels in Cushing's disease are associated with cognitive decrements. *Psychosomatic Medicine*, **63** (6), 985–993.

Statistics Sweden (2006) *Women and Men in Sweden: Facts and Figures 2006.* Statistics Sweden, Stockholm.

Statistics Sweden (2008) *Women and Men in Sweden: Facts and Figures 2008.* Statistics Sweden, Stockholm.

Steptoe, A., Cropley, M., Griffith, J. & Kirschbaum, C. (2000) Job strain and anger expression predict early morning elevations in salivary cortisol. *Psychosomatic Medicine*, **62** (2), 286–292.

Steptoe, A., Kunz-Ebrecht, S., Owen, N., *et al.* (2003a) Influence of socioeconomic status and job control on plasma fibrinogen responses to acute mental stress. *Psychosomatic Medicine*, **65** (1), 137–144.

Steptoe, A., Kunz-Ebrecht, S., Owen, N., *et al.* (2003b) Socioeconomic status and stress-related biological responses over the working day. *Psychosomatic Medicine*, **65** (3), 461–470.

Sternberg, W. (1998) Animal models of sex differences in pain and analgesia. *Journal of Musculoskeletal Pain*, **6** (3), 37–40.

Stier, H. & Lewin-Epstein, N. (2003) Time to work: A comparative analysis of preferences for working hours. *Work and Occupations*, **30** (3), 302–326.

Stockhorst, U., Steingrueber, H.J., Enck, P. & Klosterhalfen, S. (2006) Pavlovian conditioning of nausea and vomiting. *Autonomic Neuroscience – Basic & Clinical*, **129** (1–2), 50–57.

Sturm, R. & Gresenz, C.R. (2002) Relations of income inequality and family income to chronic medical conditions and mental health disorders: national survey in USA. *British Medical Journal*, **324** (7328), 20–23.

Sturman, M.C. (2003) Searching for the inverted U-shaped relationship between time and performance: meta-analyses of the experience/performance, tenure/performance, and age/performance relationships. *Journal of Management*, **29** (5), 609–640.

Su, F., Ouyang, N., Zhu, P., *et al.* (2005) Psychological stress induces chemoresistance in breast cancer by upregulating mdr1. *Biochemical and Biophysical Research Communications*, **329** (3), 888–897.

Surtees, P.G., Wainwright, N.W.J. & Khaw, K-T. (2006) Resilience, misfortune, and mortality: evidence that sense of coherence is a marker of social stress adaptive capacity. *Journal of Psychosomatic Research*, **61** (2), 221–227.

Surtees, P.G., Wainwright, N.W.J., Luben, R., Khaw, K-T. & Day, N. (2003) Sense of coherence and mortality in men and women in the EPIC-Norfolk United Kingdom Prospective Cohort Study. *American Journal of Epidemiology*, **158** (12), 1202–1209.

Suwazono, Y., Dochi, M., Sakata, K., *et al.* (2008) A longitudinal study on the effect of shift work on weight gain in male Japanese workers. *Obesity*, **16** (8), 1887–1893.

Swann, J. & Cooper, C.L. (2005) *Time Health and the Family: What Working Families Want*. A Working Families Publication, London.

Szanton, S.L., Gill, J.M. & Allen, J.K. (2005) Allostatic load: a mechanism of socioeconomic health disparities? *Biological Research for Nursing*, **7** (1), 7–15.

Tasali, E., Leproult, R., Ehrmann, D.A. & Van Cauter, E. (2008) Slow-wave sleep and the risk of type 2 diabetes in humans. *Proceedings of the National Academy of Sciences USA*, **105** (3), 1044–1049.

Taylor, S.E. (2006) Tend and befriend: biobehavioral bases of affiliation under stress. *Current Directions in Psychology Science*, **15** (6), 273–277.

Terkel, S. (1972) *Working*. Avon Books, New York.

Thaker, P.H., Han, L.Y., Kamat, A.A., *et al.* (2006) Chronic stress promotes tumor growth and angiogenesis in a mouse model of ovarian carcinoma. *Nature Medicine*, **12** (8), 939–944.

Thayer, J.F. & Lane, R.D. (2007) The role of vagal function in the risk for cardiovascular disease and mortality. *Biological Psychology*, **74** (2), 224–242.

The Economist (2005) Special report: women in business. The conundrum of the Glass Ceiling, **23**, 67–69.

Theorell, T. (eds) (2008) After 30 years with the demand–control–support model – how is it used today? *Scandinavian Journal of Work, Environment & Health* (Special Issue 6).

Toffler, A. (1970) *Future Shock*. Pan Books, London.

Tuomilehto, J., Lindström, J., Eriksson, J.G., *et al.* (2001) Prevention of type 2 diabetes mellitus by changes in lifestyle among subjects with impaired glucose tolerance. *New England Journal of Medicine*, **344** (18), 1343–1350.

Tytherleigh, M., Webb, C., Cooper, C.L. & Ricketts, C. (2005) Occupational stress in UK higher education institutions: a comparative study of all staff categories. *Higher Education Research & Development*, **24** (1), 41–61.

Uchino, B.N. (2004) *Social Support and Physical Health: Understanding the Health Consequences of Relationships*. Yale University Press, New Haven.

United Nations Children's Fund, UNICEF (2000) The State of the World's Children. Special edition. UNICEF, New York.

Ursin, H. & Eriksen, H.R. (2004) The cognitive activation theory of stress. *Psychoneuroendocrinology*, **29** (5), 567–592.

Ursin, H., Baade, E. & Levine, S. (Eds) (1978) *The Psychobiology of Stress: A Study of Coping Men*. Academic Press, New York.

US Department of Labor, Bureau of Labor Statistics, Annual Averages 2008. http://stats.bls.gov/home.htm. Last accessed 14 July 2010.

Uvnäs Moberg, K. & Pettersson, M. (2005) Oxytocin, a mediator of anti-stress, well-being, social integration, growth and healing. *Zeitschrift für Psychosomatische Medizin und Psychotherapie*, **5**, 57–80.

Vågerö, D. (2010) The East–West health divide in Europe: growing and shifting eastwards. *European Review*, **18** (1), 23–34.

Vågerö, D. & Leon, D. (1994) Effect of social class in childhood and adulthood on adult mortality. *Lancet*, **343** (8907), 1224–1225.

Van der Hulst M. (2003) Long work hours and health. *Scandinavian Journal of Work, Environment & Health*, **29** (3), 171–188.

van Doornen, L.J. & de Geus, E.J. (1989) Aerobic fitness and the cardiovascular response to stress. *Psychophysiology*, **26**, 17–28.

Van Houdenhove, B., Van Den Eede, F. & Luyten, P. (2009) Does hypothalamic–pituitary–adrenal axis hypofunction in chronic fatigue syndrome reflect a 'crash' in the stress system? *Medical Hypotheses*, **72** (6), 701–705.

Veiersted, K.B., Westgaard, R.H. & Andersen, P. (1993) Electromyographic evaluation of muscular work pattern as a predictor of trapezius myalgia. *Scandinavian Journal of Work, Environment & Health*, **19** (4), 284–290.

Verbrugge, L.M. & Wingard, D.L. (1987) Sex differentials in health and mortality. *Women and Health*, **12** (2), 103–145.

Vervoort, T., Goubert, L., Eccleston, C. Bijttebier, P. & Crombez, G. (2006) Catastrophic thinking about pain is independently associated with pain severity, disability, and somatic complaints in school children and children with chronic pain. *Journal of Pediatric Psychology*, **31** (7), 674–683.

Vingård, E., Alfredsson, L., Hagberg, M., *et al.* (2000) To what extent do current and past physical and psychosocial factors explain care-seeking for low back pain in a working population? Results from the Musculoskeletal Intervention Center-Norrtalje Study. *Spine*, **25** (4), 493–500.

Virtanen, M., Singh-Manoux, A., Ferrie, J.E., *et al.* (2009) Long working hours and cognitive function: the Whitehall II study. *American Journal of Epidemiology*, **169** (5), 596–605.

von Euler, U. & Lishajko, F. (1961) Improved technique for the fluorimetric estimation of catecholamines. *Acta Physiol. Scand*, **51**, 348–355.

von Känel, R., Bellingrath, S. & Kudielka, B.M. (2009) Overcommitment but not effort–reward imbalance relates to stress-induced coagulation changes in teachers. *Annals of Behavioral Medicine*, **37** (1), 20–28.

von Känel, R., Mills, P.J., Fainman, C. & Dimsdale, J.E. (2001) Effects of psychological stress and psychiatric disorders on blood coagulation and fibrinolysis: a biobehavioral pathway to coronary artery disease? *Psychosomatic Medicine*, **63**, 531–544.

von Thiele Schwarz, U., Lindfors, P. & Lundberg, U. (2008) Health-related effects of worksite interventions involving physical exercise and reduced workhours. *Scandinavian Journal of Work Environment & Health*, **34** (3), 179–188.

Wærsted, M. (1997) Attention-related muscle activity – a contributor to sustained occupational muscle load. PhD thesis, Department of Physiology, National Institute of Occupational Health, Oslo, Norway.

Wahlstedt, K.G.I. & Edling, C. (1997) Organizational changes at a postal sorting terminal – their effects upon work satisfaction, psychosomatic complaints and sick leave. *Work & Stress*, **11** (3), 279–291.

Wahlstedt, K.G.I., Nygård, C.H., Kemmlert, K., Togén, M. & Björkstén, M.G. (2000) The effects of a change in work organization upon the work environment and musculoskeletal symptoms among letter carriers. *International Journal of Occupational Safety and Ergonomics*, **6** (2), 237–255.

Wamala, S.P. (1999) Socioeconomic status and cardiovascular vulnerability in women. Psychosocial, behavioral and biological mediators. PhD thesis, Karolinska Institute, Stockholm.

Weber-Hamann, B., Hentschel, F., Kniest, A., *et al.* (2002) Hypercortisolemic depression is associated with increased intra-abdominal fat. *Psychosomatic Medicine,* **64** (2), 274–277.

Weinberg, A. & Cooper, C.L. (2007) *Surviving the Workplace: A Guide to Emotional Wellbeing.* Thomson, London.

Weiss, S.M. (ed.) (1981) Review Panel: Coronary-prone behavior and coronary heart disease: a critical review. *Circulation,* **63**, 1199–1215.

Wergeland, E.L., Veiersted, B., Ingre, M., *et al.* (2003) A shorter workday as a means of reducing the occurrence of musculoskeletal disorders. *Scandinavian Journal of Work, Environment & Health,* **29** (1), 27–34.

Westerlund, H., Ferrie, J.E., Hagberg, J., *et al.* (2004) Workplace expansion, long term sickness absence, and hospital admission. *Lancet,* **363** (9416), 1193–1197.

Whatmore, L., Cartwright, S. & Cooper, C.L. (1999) United Kingdom: an evaluation of a stress management programme in the public sector. In: *Preventing Stress, Improving Productivity: European Case Studies in the Workplace* (eds M. Kompier & C. Cooper). Routledge, London.

Whitehead, M., Burstrom, B. & Diderichsen, F. (1999) Social policies and the pathways to inequalities in health. A comparative analysis of lone mothers in Britain and Sweden. *Social Science and Medicine,* **50** (2), 255–270.

Wilkinson, R.G. (1992) Income distribution and life expectancy. *British Medical Journal,* **304** (6820), 165–168.

Wilkinson, R.G. (2000) *Mind the Gap: Hierarchies, Health, and Human Evolution.* Weidenfeld and Nicolson, London.

Wilkinson, R. & Pickett, K. (2009) *The Spirit Level. Why Equality is Better for Everyone.* Penguin, London.

Williams, P.G. & Thayer, J.F. (2009) Executive functioning and health: introduction to the special series. *Annals of Behavioral Medicine,* **37** (2), 101–105.

Williams, R. & Williams, V. (1994) *Anger Kills.* Harper Collins, New York.

Williams, R.B., Haney, T.L., Lee, K.L., Kong, Y.H., Blumenthal, J.A. & Whalen, R.E. (1980) Type A behavior, hostility, and coronary atherosclerosis. *Psychosomatic Medicine,* **42** (6), 539–549.

Wingenfeld, K., Wagner, D., Schmidt, I., Meinlschmidt, G., Hellhammer, D.H. & Heim, C. (2007) The low-dose dexamethasone suppression test in fibromyalgia. *Journal of Psychosomatic Research,* **62** (1), 85–91.

Wittchen, H.U., Balkau, B., Massien, C., Richard, A., Haffner, S., Pierre, J.-P., on behalf of the IDEA Steering Committee. (2006) International Day for the Evaluation of Abdominal Obesity: rationale and design of a primary care study on the prevalence of abdominal obesity and associated factors in 63 countries. *European Heart Journal* (Suppl. 8), B26–B33.

Wolf, C.J. & Salter, M.W. (2000) Neuronal plasticity: increasing the gain in pain. *Science,* **288** (5472), 1765–1769.

World Health Organization (1948) http://www.who.int/about/definition/en/print.html. Last accessed 14 July 2010.

World Health Organization (WHO) (2001) The World Health Report 2001—Mental health: New understanding, new hope. WHO, Geneva.

World Health Organization (WHO) (2006) The World Health Report 2006—Working together for health. WHO, Geneva.

Worrall, L. & Cooper, C.L. (1999) Working patterns and working hours: their impact on UK managers. *Leadership and Organization Develpoment Journal,* **20** (1), 6–10.

Worrall, L. & Cooper, C.L. (2001) Quality of Working Life Survey. Chartered Management Institute. London.

Worrall, L. & Cooper, C.L. (2007) Managers' work–life balance and health: the case of UK managers. *European Journal of International Management,* **1** (1–2), 129–145.

Worrall, L., Lindorff, M. & Cooper, C.L. (2008) Quality of Working Life 2008: A survey of organizational health and employee well-being. Comparisons of the perceptions of UK managers and managers in Victoria, Australia. Research Report, Chartered Management Institute, London.

Yusuf, S., Hawken, S., Ounpuu, S., *et al.* (2004) Effect of potentially modifiable risk factors associated with myocardial infarction in 52 countries (the INTERHEART study): case-control study. *Lancet,* **364**, 937–952.

Zoccola, P.M., Dickerson, S.S. & Lam, S. (2009) Rumination predicts longer sleep onset latency after an acute psychosocial stressor. *Psychosomatic Medicine,* **71**, 771–775.

Index

Page numbers in *italics* represent figures.

abdominal obesity   66
acute stress   60–65, 68
  alarm system   64–5
  blood coagulation   62, *78*
  digestion and energy mobilisation   63
  immune response   62
  memory and conditioning   63–4
  pain   61–2
  stage fright   65
  stress hormones   60–61
  tunnel vision   63
adaptation
  costs of   6
  general adaptation syndrome   72
  see also evolutionary perspective
adrenaline   56, 80, 93
  levels of   94
adrenocorticotrophic hormone (ACTH)   57
age and job stress   40
alarm system   64–5
alcohol   27–8
allostasis   69
allostatic load   44, 69–73, *70*,
    130, 142
anabolic processes   73–4
animals, stress in   60
antidepressants   28, 115
Antonovsky, Aaron   113
apathetic children   72–3
assembly lines   23
ASSET model   19, 111, 139
atherosclerosis   *78, 79*
attributes   55
autonomic nervous system   53–4, *54*

beliefs   55
blood coagulation   62, *78*
body mass index (BMI)   83
boundaryless jobs   30
burnout   71, 76–8

cancer   89–90
cardiovascular disease   78–9, *78*
  Baltic states   130
  gender differences   121–2
  and Type A behaviour   49–50
  see also coronary heart disease
cardiovascular system   57–8
catabolic processes   73–4
catastrophic thoughts   67
changing employment relationships   37–9
childbirth   61
children   132
  age of having   26
  contribution to workload   28
  and women's stress   128
  and workload   28
chronic fatigue   71, 76–8, *77*
chronic stress   66–8
  and neuronal death   82
Cinderella hypothesis   88, 116
circadian rhythm   117
climate change   59
Cognitive Activation Theory of Stress
    (CATS)   41, 44
cognitive function   28–9, 81–2
  conditioning   55, 63–4
  memory   63–4
  tunnel vision   63
Cohen, Sheldon   79
common cold   79–80, *80*

The Science of Occupational Health: Stress, Psychobiology and the New World of Work, first edition
By Ulf Lundberg and Cary L. Cooper. Published 2011 by Blackwell Publishing Ltd
© 2011 Ulf Lundberg and Cary L. Cooper

Keep up with critical fields

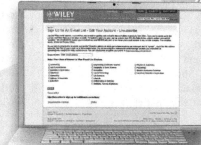

Would you like to receive up-to-date information on our books, journals and databases in the areas that interest you, direct to your mailbox?

Join the **Wiley e-mail service** - a convenient way to receive updates and exclusive discount offers on products from us.

Simply visit **www.wiley.com/email** and register online

We won't bombard you with emails and we'll only email you with information that's relevant to you. We will ALWAYS respect your e-mail privacy and NEVER sell, rent, or exchange your e-mail address to any outside company. Full details on our privacy policy can be found online.

Printed in the United States
By Bookmasters